Exploring the State of the Science of
SOLID ORGAN TRANSPLANTATION AND DISABILITY

PROCEEDINGS OF A WORKSHOP

Laura Aiuppa Denning, Megan Snair, and Ruth Cooper,
Rapporteurs

Board on Health Care Services

Health and Medicine Division

The National Academies of
SCIENCES • ENGINEERING • MEDICINE

THE NATIONAL ACADEMIES PRESS
Washington, DC
www.nap.edu

THE NATIONAL ACADEMIES PRESS   500 Fifth Street, NW   Washington, DC 20001

This activity was supported by a contract between the National Academy of Sciences and the U.S. Social Security Administration. Any opinions, findings, conclusions, or recommendations expressed in this publication do not necessarily reflect the views of any organization or agency that provided support for the project.

International Standard Book Number-13: 978-0-309-68336-4
International Standard Book Number-10: 0-309-68336-X
Digital Object Identifier: https://doi.org/10.17226/26213

Additional copies of this publication are available from the National Academies Press, 500 Fifth Street, NW, Keck 360, Washington, DC 20001; (800) 624-6242 or (202) 334-3313; http://www.nap.edu.

Copyright 2021 by the National Academy of Sciences. All rights reserved.

Printed in the United States of America

Suggested citation: National Academies of Sciences, Engineering, and Medicine. 2021. *Exploring the state of the science of solid organ transplantation and disability: Proceedings of a workshop*. Washington, DC: The National Academies Press. https://doi.org/10.17226/26213.

The National Academies of
SCIENCES · ENGINEERING · MEDICINE

The **National Academy of Sciences** was established in 1863 by an Act of Congress, signed by President Lincoln, as a private, nongovernmental institution to advise the nation on issues related to science and technology. Members are elected by their peers for outstanding contributions to research. Dr. Marcia McNutt is president.

The **National Academy of Engineering** was established in 1964 under the charter of the National Academy of Sciences to bring the practices of engineering to advising the nation. Members are elected by their peers for extraordinary contributions to engineering. Dr. John L. Anderson is president.

The **National Academy of Medicine** (formerly the Institute of Medicine) was established in 1970 under the charter of the National Academy of Sciences to advise the nation on medical and health issues. Members are elected by their peers for distinguished contributions to medicine and health. Dr. Victor J. Dzau is president.

The three Academies work together as the **National Academies of Sciences, Engineering, and Medicine** to provide independent, objective analysis and advice to the nation and conduct other activities to solve complex problems and inform public policy decisions. The National Academies also encourage education and research, recognize outstanding contributions to knowledge, and increase public understanding in matters of science, engineering, and medicine.

Learn more about the National Academies of Sciences, Engineering, and Medicine at **www.nationalacademies.org**.

The National Academies of
SCIENCES • ENGINEERING • MEDICINE

Consensus Study Reports published by the National Academies of Sciences, Engineering, and Medicine document the evidence-based consensus on the study's statement of task by an authoring committee of experts. Reports typically include findings, conclusions, and recommendations based on information gathered by the committee and the committee's deliberations. Each report has been subjected to a rigorous and independent peer-review process and it represents the position of the National Academies on the statement of task.

Proceedings published by the National Academies of Sciences, Engineering, and Medicine chronicle the presentations and discussions at a workshop, symposium, or other event convened by the National Academies. The statements and opinions contained in proceedings are those of the participants and are not endorsed by other participants, the planning committee, or the National Academies.

For information about other products and activities of the National Academies, please visit www.nationalacademies.org/about/whatwedo.

PLANNING COMMITTEE ON THE STATE OF THE SCIENCE OF SOLID ORGAN TRANSPLANTATION AND DISABILITY[1]

SARA ROSENBAUM (*Chair*), Harold and Jane Hirsh Professor, Health Law and Policy, Milken Institute School of Public Health, The George Washington University

JAMES BOWMAN, Physician, Division of Transplantation, Health Resources and Services Administration, U.S. Department of Health and Human Services

JOHN A. GOSS, Professor of Surgery, Michael E. DeBakey Department of Surgery; Chief, Division of Abdominal Transplantation, Baylor College of Medicine

PAUL L. KIMMEL, Senior Advisor, National Institute of Diabetes and Digestive and Kidney Diseases, National Institutes of Health

ERIKA D. LEASE, Medical Director, UW Lung Transplant Program; Associate Professor, Division of Pulmonary, Critical Care and Sleep Medicine; Attending Physician, Solid Organ Transplant Infectious Disease Program, University of Washington

GEORGE V. MAZARIEGOS, Chief, Pediatric Transplantation, Hillman Center for Pediatric Transplantation; Jamie Lee Curtis Endowed Chair in Transplantation Surgery, Professor of Surgery and Critical Care, University of Pittsburgh Medical Center Children's Hospital of Pittsburgh

MELISSA McQUEEN, Executive Director, Transplant Families

SHARI S. ROGAL, Assistant Professor of Medicine and Transplant Surgery, University of Pittsburgh; Physician, VA Pittsburgh Healthcare System

DORRY SEGEV, Marjory K. and Thomas Pozefsky Professor of Surgery and Epidemiology; Associate Vice Chair of Surgery; Director, Epidemiology Research Group in Organ Transplantation, Johns Hopkins University

HANNAH VALANTINE, Professor of Medicine, Division of Cardiovascular Medicine, Stanford University

---

[1] The National Academies of Sciences, Engineering, and Medicine's planning committees are solely responsible for organizing the workshop, identifying topics, and choosing speakers. The responsibility for the published Proceedings of a Workshop rests with the workshop rapporteurs and the institution.

Health and Medicine Division Staff

LAURA AIUPPA DENNING, Senior Program Officer
RUTH COOPER, Research Associate (*from January 2021*)
CYNDI TRANG, Research Associate (*until March 2021*)
RUKSHANA GUPTA, Senior Program Assistant
SHARYL NASS, Senior Director, Board on Health Care Services
JULIE WILTSHIRE, Senior Financial Business Partner

Consultant

MEGAN SNAIR, Consulting Writer

Reviewers

This Proceedings of a Workshop was reviewed in draft form by individuals chosen for their diverse perspectives and technical expertise. The purpose of this independent review is to provide candid and critical comments that will assist the National Academies of Sciences, Engineering, and Medicine in making each published proceedings as sound as possible and to ensure that it meets the institutional standards for quality, objectivity, evidence, and responsiveness to the charge. The review comments and draft manuscript remain confidential to protect the integrity of the process.

We thank the following individuals for their review of this proceedings:

YOLANDA TAI BECKER, University of Chicago
LIDA BENINSON, The National Academies of Sciences, Engineering, and Medicine
MARIO MACIS, Johns Hopkins University

Although the reviewers listed above provided many constructive comments and suggestions, they were not asked to endorse the content of the proceedings nor did they see the final draft before its release. The review of this proceedings was overseen by **KENNETH W. KIZER,** Atlas Research. He was responsible for making certain that an independent examination of this proceedings was carried out in accordance with standards of the

National Academies and that all review comments were carefully considered. Responsibility for the final content rests entirely with the rapporteurs and the National Academies.

Acknowledgments

The National Academies of Sciences, Engineering, and Medicine's Board on Health Care Services wishes to express its sincere gratitude to the planning committee chair, Sara Rosenbaum, for her valuable contributions to the development and orchestration of this workshop. The board also wishes to thank all of the members of the planning committee, who collaborated to ensure a workshop replete with informative presentations and moderated rich discussions. Finally, the board wants to thank the speakers, who generously shared their expertise and their time with workshop participants. Funding from the U.S. Social Security Administration made this workshop possible. Research assistance was provided by Christopher Lao-Scott, Senior Librarian, National Academies.

Contents

ACRONYMS AND ABBREVIATIONS   xv

1 INTRODUCTION   1
Purpose of the Workshop, 2
Organization of the Proceedings, 4

2 SOLID ORGAN TRANSPLANTATION IN THE UNITED STATES AND THE EXPERIENCES OF ORGAN RECIPIENTS AND THEIR CAREGIVERS   11
Overview of the Solid Organ Transplantation System, 11
Disparities in Transplantation Recovery and Survival, 13
Perspectives from Organ Recipients and Their Caregivers, 16
Discussion, 21

3 ORGAN TRANSPLANTATION AND DISABILITY IN ADULTS   25
Clinical Conditions and Consequences for Health and Function, 25
Discussion, 32
Assessing Physical, Cognitive, and Psychosocial Function in Adults After Organ Transplantation, 34
Discussion, 39

4 ORGAN TRANSPLANTATION AND DISABILITY IN CHILDREN AND ADOLESCENTS 43
Clinical Conditions and Consequences for Health and Function, 43
Adolescent Transitions to Adulthood After Transplantation, 53
Discussion, 55
Assessing Physical, Cognitive, and Psychosocial Function After Organ Transplantation in Children, 57
Discussion, 60

5 TREATMENTS, TECHNOLOGIES, AND INTERVENTIONS AFFECTING FUNCTION AFTER TRANSPLANTATION 63
Pretransplant Care Management, 63
Pharmacologic Treatments After Transplantation, 66
Rehabilitation After Transplantation, 68
Palliative Care, 70
Discussion, 73

6 FUTURE OUTLOOK FOR ORGAN TRANSPLANTATION AND DISABILITY 77
COVID-19-Related Concerns for Transplant Patients, 78
Emerging Technologies to Watch, 80
Final Thoughts, 81

REFERENCES 83

APPENDIXES
A STATEMENT OF TASK 93
B WORKSHOP AGENDA 95
C BIOGRAPHICAL SKETCHES OF WORKSHOP PLANNING COMMITTEE MEMBERS AND SPEAKERS 101

Boxes, Figures, and Table

BOXES

1-1 Key Points by Individual Speakers and Participants, 5

3-1 Interventions for Clinicians to Assist Recipients in Return to Work, 40

5-1 Definition of Palliative Care, 71
5-2 Elements of Palliative Care and Common Outcomes, 71

FIGURES

2-1 Levels of racism relevant to each level of the social ecology, 14
2-2 Factors that influence disparities in access to care and quality of health care services, by level, 15

3-1 Summary of contributing factors leading to frailty, 35

4-1 Hierarchy of outcome measures, 45
4-2 Pediatric liver transplantation across three tiers of outcomes, 46
4-3 Pediatric intestine transplantation across three tiers of outcomes, 47
4-4 Functional status of surviving pediatric lung transplant recipients, 51

5-1 Three components of the strength training interventions for liver transplant patients based on the Information-Motivation-Behavioral Skills conception model for modifying individual health behaviors, 64

5-2 Brain function and metabolism in patients with long-term tacrolimus therapy after kidney transplantation compared to patients after liver transplantation and healthy controls, 67

TABLE

2-1 Percent Patient and Graft Survival, Return to Work, and Quality of Life (QOL) 1 Year After Transplantation by Organ Type, 13

Acronyms and Abbreviations

CF	cystic fibrosis
CHD	congenital heart disease
CKD	chronic kidney disease
CLAD	chronic lung allograft dysfunction
CMV	cytomegalovirus
COPD	chronic obstructive pulmonary disease
EPTS	estimated posttransplant survival score
ESRD	end-stage renal disease
HCV	hepatitis C virus
ICU	intensive care unit
JHU	Johns Hopkins University
KDPI	kidney donor profile index
KDRI	kidney donor risk index
MELD	model for end-stage liver disease
MRI	magnetic resonance imaging

OPTN	Organ Procurement and Transplantation Network
PedsQL	Pediatric Quality of Life Inventory Tool
PKD	polycystic kidney disease
PTSD	posttraumatic stress disorder
SRTR	Scientific Registry of Transplant Recipients
SSA	U.S. Social Security Administration
UNOS	United Network for Organ Sharing
QOL	quality of life

1

Introduction[1]

Transplantation of a solid organ, such as a kidney, heart, or liver, is a lifesaving procedure and is sometimes the only viable treatment for patients experiencing end-stage organ failure as a result of illness or injury. A growing prevalence of solid organ diseases in the United States is contributing to an increasing number of people needing a transplant and longer wait times on the national transplant waiting list. New scientific knowledge and technologies are showing improved survival rates and other benefits to patients, giving reason for optimism. However, while transplantation can lengthen a person's life, the road to recovery is difficult and complex. While some transplant recipients are able to return to a more active life, others experience greater functional limitations due to health factors, medication side effects, organ rejection, or other setbacks, making it difficult for adults to return to work and for children to do well developmentally and across various domains of functioning.

To gain an understanding of current scientific findings in the field of solid organ transplantation, the U.S. Social Security Administration (SSA)

---

[1] The planning committee's role was limited to planning the workshop, and the Proceedings of a Workshop was prepared by the workshop rapporteurs as a factual summary of what occurred at the workshop. Statements, recommendations, and opinions expressed are those of individual presenters and participants and are not necessarily endorsed or verified by the National Academies of Sciences, Engineering, and Medicine, and they should not be construed as reflecting any group consensus.

asked the National Academies of Sciences, Engineering, and Medicine's (the National Academies') Board on Health Care Services to organize a virtual public workshop to examine disability associated with organ transplantation. As part of its charge, SSA asked the National Academies to focus on the functional outcomes for adults and children who are solid organ transplant recipients and to facilitate discussions related to the following topics:

- Processes conducted to identify transplant recipients with the highest probability of positive posttransplantation outcomes;
- Current outcome measures for assessing effectiveness of care for individuals who have undergone organ transplantation (e.g., morbidity and mortality);
- Treatments used to improve a person's physical or mental functioning following organ transplantation and the settings in which the treatments are provided;
- The typical length of time from transplant surgery until the person's functioning improves to the point of which their condition is no longer disabling, and specific ages or other recipient traits where improvement is more likely;
- Laboratory or other findings used to assess medical and functional improvement after organ transplant; and
- Recent medical advances or new technologies that may improve expected patient outcomes, and potential advances anticipated in the near future.

The workshop focused on kidney, heart, liver, and lung transplantation, and to a lesser extent, intestine transplantation. The workshop planning committee invited subject-matter experts to present on important aspects of posttransplantation recovery and functioning in adults and children. The workshop was held virtually on March 22–23, 2021. This Proceedings of a Workshop describes the speakers' presentations and the moderated panel discussions, which included panelists' responses to questions from SSA staff in the audience and from the general public.

PURPOSE OF THE WORKSHOP

In the opening remarks, Sara Rosenbaum, professor of health law and policy at The George Washington University and chair of the workshop planning committee, described the purpose of the workshop as translational. As SSA is tasked with the responsibility of translating medical knowledge into policies and practices when evaluating disability claims, she explained, it needs the most current and comprehensive research to do so. This exploration can also help it understand what organ transplantation recovery looks like in comparison to recovery from other conditions that lead to functional limitations and to place organ transplantation recovery within the broader context of the SSA disability program.

From SSA, Gina Clemons, associate commissioner of the Office of Disability Policy, and Vincent Nibali, policy analyst for the Office of Medical Policy, explained the reasons for the workshop and gave a brief overview of the disability process. Clemons stated that the information addressed by the workshop is needed to help SSA ensure that its criteria for evaluating disability claims of organ transplant recipients are up to date with new scientific findings in the field. She said SSA is interested in information about the nature of recovery after transplantation and the different ways that disability may persist. For example, a patient may have recovered from a transplant but continues to experience side effects from treatment or comorbid conditions. Clemons said that knowing how these issues can manifest when both evaluating and re-evaluating patient functional status will help SSA make more informed decisions on disability benefits.

Nibali stated that Congress defines disability in adults as "the inability to engage in substantial gainful activity by reason of a medically determinable physical or mental impairment or combination of impairments, which is expected to last for a continuous period of not less than 12 months or result in death"[2] and in children as "marked and severe functional limitations." When SSA determines if a claimant is disabled based on the severity of functional limitations, it compares those functional limitations with the current medical criteria[3] that apply to its evaluation of impairments. Thus, Nibali explained, it is crucial that SSA has a complete and comprehensive

---

[2] The definition of disability is described in Section 223(d)(1) of the Social Security Act as an "inability to engage in any substantial gainful activity by reason of any medically determinable physical or mental impairment which can be expected to result in death or which has lasted or can be expected to last for a continuous period of not less than 12 months, or in the case of an individual who has attained the age of 55 and is blind (within the meaning of blindness as defined in section 216(i)(1)), inability by reason of such blindness to engage in substantial gainful activity requiring skills or abilities comparable to those of any gainful activity in which the individual has previously engaged with some regularity and over a substantial period of time" (Social Security Act, 42 U.S.C. § 423(d)).

[3] SSA refers to these medical criteria as the Listing of Impairments.

understanding of the criteria that may constitute functional impairment in organ transplant recipients to ensure they meet the threshold for benefits.

ORGANIZATION OF THE PROCEEDINGS

This proceedings is organized into six chapters. Following the introduction, Chapter 2 presents an overview of solid organ transplantation in the United States and experiences of patients and caregivers. Chapter 3 covers the various types of transplantation in adults and ways to assess functioning, while Chapter 4 focuses on the pediatric and adolescent transplant population. Various treatments and technologies that can affect functioning are discussed in Chapter 5; and finally, Chapter 6 reflects on the presentations and provides commentary on potential future implications for the solid organ transplant field. Appendix A includes the Statement of Task for the workshop. Appendixes B and C provide the workshop agenda and short biographical sketches of the workshop planning committee members and speakers, respectively. The speakers' presentations and the webcast have been archived online.[4]

Box 1-1 summarizes key points from speakers and participants during the workshop.

---

[4] See https://www.nationalacademies.org/event/03-22-2021/the-state-of-the-science-on-organ-transplantation-and-disability-a-workshop-part-1 (accessed May 6, 2021).

BOX 1-1
Key Points by Individual Speakers and Participants[a]

Perspectives on the Organ Transplantation System
- The rising rates of solid organ diseases in the United States are contributing to greater morbidity, mortality, and need for transplants. The demand for the organs far exceeds supply. (Mulligan)
- The benefits of organ transplantation are many and may include increased life expectancy, improved quality of life (QOL), maintaining independence, and the ability to return to work, but every patient is unique, and there can be many obstacles to successful transplantation outcomes. (Lease, Mulligan, Purnell, Rogal)
- The benefits of transplantation are not equal for all recipients; outcomes have racial, ethnic, and economic disparities. Greater gaps in disparities appear in the data at 5–10 years after transplant. (Purnell)
- The fragmented U.S. health system requires high levels of case coordination that can leave patients vulnerable to gaps in care during the handoffs across systems. (Bowman)
- Children who are transitioning to adult-focused care are highly at risk of adverse outcomes, yet fewer than half of these special needs patients, including pediatric transplant recipients, receive adequate support and services for that transition. (Diaz-Gonzalez de Ferris)
- Patient and graft survival rates are the most common metrics used to report transplant success, as transplant centers are held accountable for these metrics up until 1 year afterward. While transplantation is a lifesaving treatment, most recipients experience significant morbidity. Underlying conditions, hospitalizations, surgeries and procedures, immunosuppressive medications, and other treatments all contribute to adverse effects and limitations on daily activities. (Chin, Lease, Mazariegos, Montgomery, Rogal, Segev)
- At 3 and 5 years after transplantation, data show a strong majority of adult patients in all organ transplant types report good QOL, but at 5 years after transplantation, between 40 to 60 percent of patients still have not returned to work, with kidney patients being the most likely to do so and lung patients the least. (Mulligan)

continued

BOX 1-1 Continued

- Transplantation treats organ failure; it does not address many of the physical, mental, and personal reasons that could lead to needing a transplant, such as diabetes or substance abuse disorders, which can affect recovery and lead to poor outcomes. (Rogal)
- System barriers to success in the early posttransplant phase include the scarcity of available rehabilitation programs; in addition, insurers often do not cover the rehabilitation required, and many patients are unable to pay out of pocket. (Patel)
- Data on posttransplant functioning are lacking in transplant registries, and the data have gaps on race, wealth, sex, and mental health. (Kimmel, Purnell, Valantine)
- Systemic effects of COVID-19 are unknown at this time, but studies are under way to examine the safety of transplants for people who tested positive for COVID-19 and the safety of using organs from donors who tested positive. Vaccine effectiveness in transplant recipients is also being investigated. (A. Gupta, Lease, Patel)
- Returning to work during the COVID-19 pandemic also illuminates key questions about protections in place for recipients who want to contribute to society. (Purnell)

Clinical and Functional Outcomes in Adults
- Some major factors affecting transplant outcomes include etiology, age, pretransplant status, underlying conditions and comorbidities, frailty, exercise capacity, medical contraindications, and donor factors. (Conrad, Lease, Rogal, Segev, Valantine)
- Posttransplant survival can be predicted on the basis of clinical indicators (such as the model for end-stage liver disease [MELD] scores for liver transplants and the estimated posttransplant survival score [EPTS] for kidney transplants), but the factors associated with posttransplant function are less well established. (Rogal, Segev)
- Kidney patients with an EPTS score of 0–20 percent had a 90 percent survival rate at 10 years after transplantation, whereas patients with a score of 81–100 percent had only a 40 percent survival rate. (Segev)
- Liver transplant survival rates are very high, with 86 percent still alive at 1 year after transplantation and 72 percent at 5 years after transplantation. (Rogal)

- Long-term survival rates in lung transplantation are limited and have not changed much in recent years despite strides in surgical techniques and posttransplant care. Cystic fibrosis patients have the best survival rates, at almost 10 years. (Lease)
- Overall survival following a heart transplant is 91 percent at 1 year, and at 5 years, it is 75 percent. Patients with mechanical support of the heart before transplant are less likely to fully rehabilitate and regain maximum function after transplantation. (Valantine)
- Even with successful transplants, the vast majority of patients experience life-changing deficits in physical, cognitive, and psychosocial functioning that often result in needing frequent medical and supportive care over their lifetime. (Edwards, Hoyt-Trapp, Keefer, McQueen, Montgomery, Thomas, Vlahos)
- Studies show that transplant recipients show some improvement in QOL following transplant, but the level is more comparable to other patients with chronic disease than to the levels of healthy people. (DiMartini)
- Cognitive impairment is highly prevalent in recipients. (A. Gupta)
- Frailty in pretransplant patients is common and associated with a higher risk of mortality, hospital readmissions, and declines in posttransplant physical, psychosocial, and cognitive function. (McAdams-DeMarco, Patel, Segev)
- Prehabilitation (pretransplant care management), rehabilitation, and palliative care have demonstrated benefits and improved outcomes for transplant candidates and recipients, and more patients would benefit from their wider use and availability. (Mathur, McAdams-DeMarco, Wentlandt)
- The research evidence supporting interventions is strongest for heart transplants, where cardiac rehabilitation has been shown to significantly improve functional capacity, QOL, and cognition—and translate into long-term benefits. Cardiac rehabilitation is now a routine part of care but less so for other organs, where the evidence is less established. (Patel)
- Pharmacological strategies to improve functioning include limiting corticosteroids, recognizing and treating mental health disorders, regulating levels of anti-rejection medications, and monitoring long term for hypertension, diabetes, and malignancy. (Mohammad)

continued

BOX 1-1 Continued

Factors Affecting Return to Work
- Many factors are responsible for the disparities between recipients' reports of a positive QOL and their ability to return to work, including the fear of losing disability benefits or health care coverage, which would threaten access to critical medications; challenges associated with mental health problems, including depression and substance use disorders; an aging transplant population nearing retirement; the fear of unsafe working conditions with greater exposure to viruses or infections; and a general lack of employee protections and accommodations, such as time off for rigorous follow-up appointments and ongoing care. (Lease, Patel, Purnell, Rogal, Thomas)
- Studies show that decisions regarding return to work are also influenced by education level, depression levels, and pretransplant employment status. The longer one is unemployed before transplantation, the longer it would take to be employed after. (Thomas)
- Achieving the levels of functioning that returning to work entails in large part depends on the availability of essential services and supports. (DiMartini, Rogal, Valantine)
- For many, struggles with adverse consequences just get started at 1 year after transplantation, but that is often where recipients really start to feel a sudden void in services and support. (Montgomery)

Clinical Outcomes and Functioning in Children
- More than 27,000 children are living with a functional allograft in the United States today, with liver and kidney transplants being the highest, compared to fewer heart and significantly fewer intestine and lung recipients. (Mazariegos)
- Pediatric liver transplant recipients fare significantly better in terms of graft outcomes than those requiring intestine transplants. Only about 25 percent of liver recipients using deceased donors had graft failure after 10 years after transplantation, compared to 40–60 percent of intestine recipients. (Mazariegos)
- Compared to adults with end-stage kidney disease, children with this disease fare much better and have 10-year survival rates of 85–90 percent. (Diaz-Gonzalez de Ferris)
- Half-lives for adolescent heart transplant patients were quite similar to adults, around 14–15 years, compared to babies, who have much higher half-lives of 25 years. Even 5 years after trans-

plant, 30 percent of pediatric patients are rehospitalized due to rejection and infection. (Chin)
- Pediatric lung transplants are very rare and patients currently have a median survival of 9.1 years, but survival has been improving since 2010. (Conrad)
- Physical functioning is closest to normal in pediatric liver and kidney recipients, but heart transplant recipients are the most at risk for cognitive impairments because of lower oxygen levels. (Mohammad)
- Rehabilitation and physical therapy help pediatric lung transplant patients achieve normal activities in their lives, including school, sports, and good physical, social, and mental health outcomes. (Conrad)
- Taking immunosuppressive medications from early on in life for many years can have adverse effects on the developing brain. (Mohammad)
- During the transition from pediatric to adult care, adolescents are at great risk of nonadherence to medication regimens and provider visits, which results in higher rates of rejection and other poor outcomes. (Diaz-Gonzalez de Ferris, N. Gupta, Shemesh)
- Transplantation during childhood can have significant consequences on functioning in adulthood; barriers to care, a scarce number of specialized programs, and the lack of age-appropriate support services can hinder successful functioning. (Chin, Diaz-Gonzalez de Ferris, N. Gupta, Shemesh)

Views on Improving Success in Transplantation
- It is necessary to improve and gauge which interventions promote positive long-term outcomes following a transplant that go beyond just measuring survival and instead focus on the individual's needs and QOL. (Conrad, N. Gupta, Lease, Mathur, Mohammad, Montgomery)
- Transitioning to a more holistic standard when viewing outcomes metrics is particularly important in the pediatric population, as their cycle of care is measured in decades, compared to years for adults. (Mazariegos)
- Better metrics are needed to assess and track outcomes and identify modifiable factors in physical and cognitive functioning. More age-appropriate and disease-specific measures of functioning and greater use of real-time assessments using technologies such as activity trackers or wearable devices would be beneficial. (Mohammad, Patel)

continued

BOX 1-1 Continued

- To combat transplant inequalities, various interventions are needed that target recipients, families, providers, and communities, including patient education, programs to ensure affordability of care, and policy changes in the transplant system. (Purnell)
- Dedicated case management can improve the challenges individual transplant patients experience. (Bowman)
- Targeted culturally and cognitively appropriate patient education and engagement interventions can lead to improved health care transitions and self-management among adolescents. (Diaz-Gonzalez de Ferris, A. Gupta)
- Improved screening and early treatment of mental health issues are critical to successful recovery and return to work following transplant. (DiMartini)
- Further research in the areas of prehabilitation, rehabilitation, and palliative care is needed to create multidisciplinary approaches that target the spectrum of needs of specific patients and provide optimal regimens and delivery modes. Assessing the impacts on long-term survival, QOL, and other posttransplant outcomes and reducing clinician barriers to these services are other important areas of research. (Mathur, McAdams-DeMarco, Wentlandt)

[a] This list is the rapporteurs' summary of points made by the individual speakers identified, and the statements have not been endorsed or verified by the National Academies of Sciences, Engineering, and Medicine. They are not intended to reflect a consensus among workshop participants.

2

Solid Organ Transplantation in the United States and the Experiences of Organ Recipients and Their Caregivers

Solid organ transplantation is a lifesaving procedure for many patients with end-stage organ failure. While the cutting-edge research, best practices, and evidence-based treatments can contribute a large amount of knowledge to the field, many workshop speakers reminded the audience that patients are at the center of the discourse about posttransplantation recovery and functioning. This chapter summarizes presentations and discussions from the first and third workshop sessions. Speakers in the first session provided an overview of the U.S. transplantation system, including how organs are donated and allocated, the availability of organs, outcome data, and disparities in the recovery and survival rates. Patients, a caregiver, and a social worker in the third session conveyed what it is like to live with an organ transplant.

OVERVIEW OF THE SOLID ORGAN TRANSPLANTATION SYSTEM

Opening the first session, David Mulligan, president of the Organ Procurement and Transplantation Network (OPTN) and the United Network for Organ Sharing (UNOS), began by discussing how solid organ diseases, such as chronic kidney disease (CKD) or cardiomyopathy, which can result in the need for a transplant, are more common than most people think and that demand far exceeds supply. Mulligan introduced two methods of organ donation: living donation and deceased donation. Living donors may either donate via direct donation to a specific recipient or act as a non-direct "Good Samaritan" donor where the recipient is unknown. Kidney donors may also donate via paired donation, where a family member may wish to donate a kidney to a relative, but their blood type is incompatible. When this situation occurs, the related donor may instead donate to a nonrelated recipient in exchange for a kidney from a family member of that recipient, resulting in a "kidney swap." The second method is deceased donation. Deceased donors may be considered either brain dead, characterized by no brain stem function, or experiencing circulatory death. Mulligan noted that while the number of organ transplants from deceased donors is growing, there is still a shortage of all solid organs.

OPTN, which maintains the national transplant list, plays an important role in living donation by maintaining quality standards and requirements through guidelines for donor evaluation and informed consent. It also provides training for the personnel in living donor programs. Together, Mulligan noted, OPTN and UNOS maintain a national database of available organs and the transplant waiting list and help to distribute organs equitably based on a set list of matching criteria, such as medical urgency, blood type, organ size, waiting time, and geographic distance. Mulligan discussed the survival rates for transplant patients. Table 2-1 highlights the survival rates for patients and grafts for all organ types 1 year after transplantation. Using OPTN data from 2015–2019, Mulligan discussed how despite 70–80 percent of patients having a high-performance status[1] across all organ types, few are able to return to income-generating work. He noted that when looking at long-term data, such as 3 and 5 years after transplantation, the outcomes are similar: a strong majority of patients in all organ transplant types report good quality of life (QOL), but at 5 years after transplantation, 40–60 percent still have not returned to work, with kidney patients being the most likely and lung patients the least. Mulligan explained that 16 to 27 percent of patients do not have a reported performance status at 5 years after transplantation and beyond, meaning that while it is known whether these patients are still living, their QOL and return-to-work status remain unknown. Mulligan concluded by stating that

---

[1] Performance status is a numerical rating of a patient's ability to perform normal activities, including the ability to care for oneself (getting dressed, eating, and bathing) and to engage in more vigorous activity (cleaning a house, working at a job). The Karnofsky scale (100–0) is widely used. A normal score is between 80–100 percent (see Karnofsky et al., 1948).

TABLE 2-1 Percent Patient and Graft Survival, Return to Work, and Quality of Life (QOL) 1 Year After Transplantation by Organ Type

	Kidney	Liver	Heart	Lung
Patient Survival (%)	96	94	91	89
Graft Survival (%)	94	92	90	89
Return to Work (%)	31	21	21	14
Normal QOL (%)	75	72	80	70

NOTE: Normal QOL is defined by a Karnofsky score of 80–100 percent.
SOURCES: Adapted from David Mulligan presentation, March 22, 2021. Based on Organ Procurement and Transplantation Network (OPTN) data, including transplants from January 1, 2015, to December 31, 2019.

while solid organ transplants have become increasingly successful, the rising rates of solid organ diseases in the United States is contributing to greater morbidity, mortality, and need for transplants.

DISPARITIES IN TRANSPLANTATION RECOVERY AND SURVIVAL

Tanjala Purnell, associate director of the Johns Hopkins Center for Health Equity and Urban Health Institute, has conducted extensive research on topics such as racial, ethnic, and wealth disparities in transplant recovery and survival. She framed her talk by stating that many factors contribute to differing transplant survival rates, such as age, body mass index, and etiology, as discussed in Chapter 3; but she said many social factors also contribute to whether transplant outcomes are positive or negative. She discussed the extensive benefits of transplantation, such as increased life expectancy, better QOL, maintaining independence, and the ability to return to work (Purnell et al., 2013). Purnell emphasized that the benefits, however, are not equal for all transplant recipients. Racial and ethnic disparities in heart transplant outcomes exist: Asian Americans have the highest graft survival rates, while African Americans have the lowest (Morris et al., 2016). Poverty levels and sex are also indicative of transplant outcomes, specifically graft survival. When examining 5-year kidney transplant outcomes, data show no significant difference in graft survival for men and women who live in wealthy neighborhoods, but as poverty levels increase, women are more likely to experience graft failure (Purnell et al., 2019). Nevertheless, kidney transplant outcomes tell an encouraging story. Purnell et al. (2016b) conducted a study of racial disparities in kidney transplant outcomes spanning two decades and found increasingly similar survival rates between African American and White patients.

To understand racial, ethnic, and economic disparities in transplant outcomes, Purnell emphasized that examining the root cause is key, and stated that disparities exist because of multiple factors, including systemic racism. Arriola (2017) proposed a model of different types of racism experienced by African American transplant recipients, including internalized racism, personally mediated racism, and institutionalized racism (see Figure 2-1). Institutionalized racism is the largest portion of the model, presenting as institutionalized factors, community factors, and public policy. Purnell indicated that structural racism is another form and defined it as the mechanisms by which societies foster racial discrimination through systems of housing, education, employment, earnings, benefits, credit, media, health care, and criminal justice that reinforce discriminatory beliefs, values, and distribution of resources (Bailey et al., 2017). She showed data from the Baltimore City Health Department (Barbot, 2014) as an example

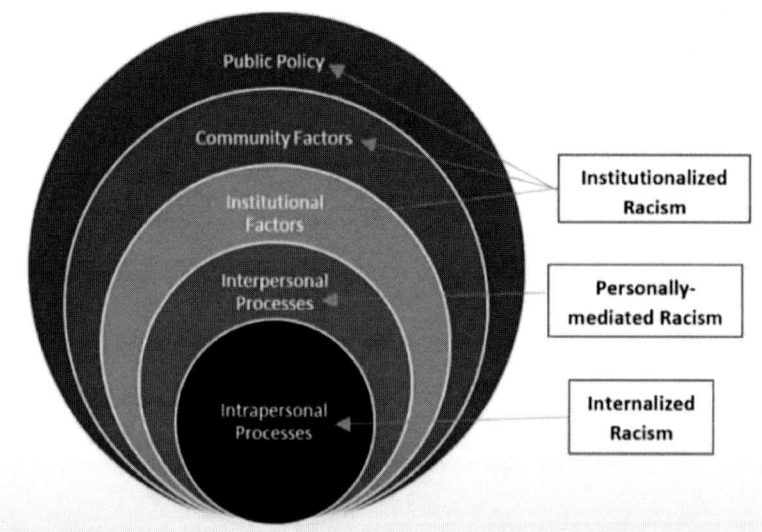

FIGURE 2-1 Levels of racism relevant to each level of the social ecology.
SOURCES: Tanjala Purnell presentation, March 22, 2021; Arriola, Kimberly Jacob. "Race, Racism, and Access to Renal Transplantation Among African Americans." *Journal of Health Care for the Poor and Underserved* 28:1 (2017), 35, Figure 1. © 2017 Meharry Medical College. Reprinted with permission of Johns Hopkins University Press.

of a practice called "redlining" (a form of residential segregation) and she explained that such institutionalized practices contribute to the economic and racial inequalities seen in organ transplant outcomes.

Purnell ended her presentation by posing the question of what needs to be done from a policy standpoint to achieve better transplant outcomes. She explained there is already general awareness of inequalities, such as patients from poorer neighborhoods experiencing worse outcomes, and so what is needed now is a targeted, multilevel approach to combat transplant inequalities. Purnell et al. (2016a) suggested intervention techniques designed to target individual patients as well as families, providers, and communities, ranging from patient education to programs to ensure affordability of care, to policy changes (see Figure 2-2). Her multilevel approach aims at improving clinical outcomes, avoiding hospital readmissions, improving the patient care experience, and ensuring equity of services. Despite a few encouraging statistics showing that the racial inequality gaps in transplant outcomes may be getting smaller, there is still a long way to go to combat racial, ethnic, and wealth disparities in transplant outcomes, she concluded.

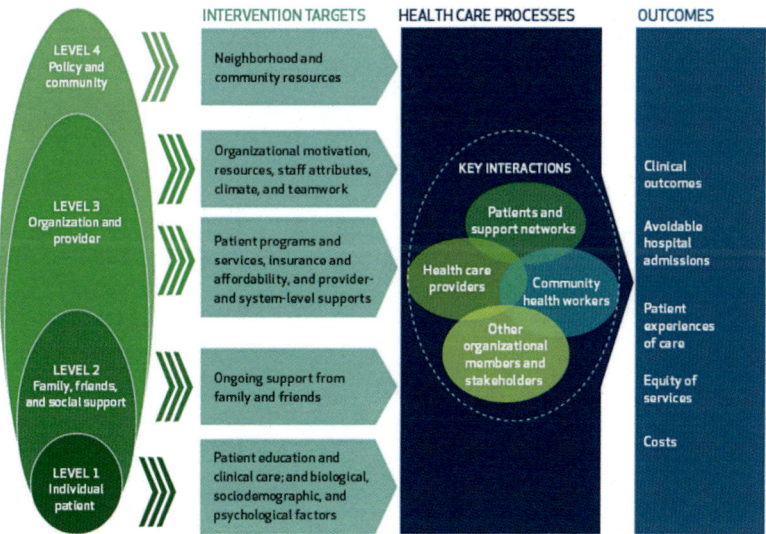

FIGURE 2-2 Factors that influence disparities in access to care and quality of health care services, by level.
SOURCES: Tanjala Purnell presentation, March 22, 2021; Purnell et al., 2016a.

PERSPECTIVES FROM ORGAN RECIPIENTS AND THEIR CAREGIVERS

An understanding of transplantation recovery and functioning cannot be attained by only looking at the transplantation system and policies or merely reviewing the science. The picture would be incomplete without the stories about the realities of life as told by people needing a transplant, people living with a transplant, or their caregivers. This section offers several first-person perspectives from organ recipients and then highlights a caregiver's perspective and the viewpoint of a social worker who is paired with patients during and after a transplant.

Organ Recipient Perspectives

Five adults who had undergone organ transplantations shared stories about their journeys and what life is like now in the years after the procedure. They discussed the challenges of living with chronic diseases and the difficulties of managing life after organ transplantation.

Valen Keefer described her transplant journey beginning at the age of 10, when she was diagnosed with polycystic kidney disease (PKD), a hereditary disease that has taken the lives of many of her family members. Keefer said PKD caused pain and required many hospital stays as a child and a year-long stay in college. She finally had both kidneys removed, underwent 7 months of dialysis, and eventually received a kidney transplant at the age of 19. Keefer emphasized that she had a long road to recovery, which included taking 40 pills per day, dealing with side effects, and getting sick often because of her suppressed immune system. "While the transplant gave me a second chance at life, it didn't cure my disease," Keefer said. "Fourteen years following the kidney transplant, I got severely ill again," she explained, "and after numerous recurrent sepsis episodes and daily antibiotics, I needed a lifesaving liver transplant." Receiving an organ transplant is a singular event that does not translate into being fine once the procedure is over, she noted, and it requires dedication and resilience and is quite exhausting, both physically and mentally. "I've been a patient my whole life," Keefer continued, "not knowing how I'm going to feel day to day. A fever or single lab number being off could lead to hospital stays." She stressed the difficulty of being in her late 30s and still unable to maintain a full-time job, but added that she strives to take the best care of her health she can in order to be a contributing member to society, in gratitude to organ donors, and as an advocate for the transplant community.

Dawn Edwards introduced herself as a kidney transplant patient; she had kidney disease for 29 years and underwent a transplant in 2003 after 10 years on dialysis. Her journey was difficult from the start, she said. She was released 5 days after receiving her transplant, but had to go back daily for routine infusions. Then, 10 days later, she had her first rejection episode, which was "completely frightening," but doctors were able to control it. During that episode, they discovered that she had acquired cytomegalovirus (CMV) from her donor. In addition to surgery recovery, Edwards shared that she also had a lot of stomach and intestinal problems from CMV. She described the first 3 years after transplantation like a roller coaster, and she was often in the hospital with either colitis or a rejection episode. But, she said, she always thought she would go back to work when the 3 years of disability benefits were up, so she had to focus on getting better in that time. She acknowledged that she could not return to her previous job because of the physical demands, so she thought about how to reinvent herself. Still, throughout this time, she continued to have episodes that made her recovery very difficult. She experienced side effects from anti-rejection medications, such as osteoporosis, which led to a broken hip that needed to be replaced after stepping off a curb one day. Edwards said that things started to settle down after the third year, and she was lucky to be offered a position within her end-stage renal disease (ESRD) network as her disability benefits ended. She attempted a trial period at the position; she still had occasional hospitalizations, but it went well, and her employer was very understanding. "I think disability for people with kidney transplants needs to be individualized," Edwards stated; "it can't just be the recovery from journey in and of itself." She added that many patients would feel more comfortable if they did not have the pressure of needing to go back to work after that 3-year period or risk losing their health care coverage.

Stephanie Hoyt-Trapp was diagnosed with nonalcoholic steatohepatitis, an advanced form of nonalcoholic fatty liver disease, about 10 years ago. Six years ago, she explained, she had to have a transplant because her liver had essentially ceased functioning. She was forced to stop her practice as a clinical psychologist and had just adopted an infant a few years prior as a single parent. She had many responsibilities but suddenly could not handle any of them and had to go on disability. "Getting a transplant was obviously the hardest thing I've ever done," Hoyt-Trapp said. "Prior to the procedure I was very upbeat and positive that things were going to be okay." She went on to say that she had thought she would return to her normal life, but when she did not, it was a huge turning point. Separate from the physical challenges, she explained, her biggest challenge was her level of depression. She tried going through rehabilitation, but it did not help, and being unable to work, she said it felt like she was not doing anything of value. Finally, she shared, just recently she was asked to participate as a subject-matter expert on a research grant related to pain and cirrhosis. She said the work has allowed her to feel useful, use her brain, and have a valued opinion. "Having that sense of worth does a lot to help you get through this," she added.

Sharing her perspective as a lung transplant recipient, Fanny Vlahos introduced herself as a licensed attorney, as well as many other roles including mother, who was born with cystic fibrosis (CF), a disease that mostly affects the lungs and pancreas. When she was born, the life expectancy for someone with CF was 14, Vlahos shared, but she recently celebrated her 40th birthday. She acknowledged that she is here today because she received a lifesaving double lung transplant 9 years ago. While she was fortunate and only mildly affected with CF for most of her life, she contracted pneumonia while pregnant and went from 130 percent lung function to needing a lung transplant in just 14 months, receiving new lungs when her baby was 10 months old. When thinking of going back to work, Vlahos explained, she had to consider her weekly doctor appointments, routine procedures, dozens of daily medications, and sensitivities to things in the environment that could compromise her suppressed immune system. She knew the legal community could not be as flexible as she needed, and had to stop her career and become a stay-at-home mom. Throughout her recovery, she endured both routine complications and near-fatal setbacks, with numerous gastrointestinal complications due to anti-rejection medications. Some days, Vlahos said she feels strong and ready to conquer the world, and other days, she feels her body is failing her, emphasizing that both the physical and mental stressors that come with this life are now her new normal. While her family has been with her through this entire journey, she pointed out that it is difficult for others—especially hiring managers—to understand her circumstances, because she looks "healthy" on the outside. But, living as a transplant patient has no finish line, and she said it is more than a full-time job to maintain her health. She wishes that employers would consider her value as a competent attorney with two law degrees, not as a liability for being an organ transplant recipient.

Robert Montgomery is a transplant surgeon at the New York University Langone Medical Center who also underwent a heart transplant. He has had a genetic heart disease, familial dilated cardiomyopathy, his whole life, but it became progressively worse. Though he was diagnosed early in his career as a resident, he was able to continue for years as a transplant surgeon. In 2018, his condition acutely worsened, and he became very ill, ending up in the ICU in an urgent situation. He noted that he was lucky to receive a heart, but his donor had died from a drug overdose and had hepatitis C virus (HCV) infection, requiring Montgomery to take additional medication to clear the virus from his blood. His recovery was fairly rapid, but he found himself facing new challenges that he did not anticipate, even after seeing thousands of transplant patients in his career. Most challenges were related to side effects from drugs—especially a tremor from one particular drug. While most patients just get used to it, he said, that is really not an option for a surgeon. So he spent a long time searching for an alternative drug that would not cause tremors. Montgomery reiterated the comments of other speakers, saying that you do not simply return to your normal life after a transplant. Instead, you take on a whole new challenge of being immunocompromised, which has significant risks and pitfalls. Fortunately, he admitted, he has been able to return fully to work as a surgeon and administrator, but he noted it has not been an easy journey.

Caregiver Perspective

For some patients, especially young children, the caregiver's role can be just as challenging as the patients themselves. Melissa McQueen from Transplant Families shared her experience as a mother and caregiver when her son had to undergo a heart transplant as a baby. She shared that he nearly died right after birth and then was diagnosed with dilated cardiomyopathy. McQueen's son was eventually able to leave the hospital, but the treatments were not enough, and by the time he was 8 months old, he needed a heart transplant. Because they did not have a transplant center close to their home, they had to fly to Dallas, Texas, and were able to receive a heart shortly after the initial evaluation. Afterward, she said, he was a whole new baby, ready to tackle life. While they had hoped that would be the end of their journey, McQueen said in reality it was not. Many families do not talk about the difficult recovery, she said, and shared stories about some of the many stays in the hospital as he got older. He suffered from immune suppression problems and *clostridium difficile* infection and had to navigate many years of speech and occupational therapy. He also missed many milestones in early childhood. She said it was very difficult to get back on track after that and commented on the challenges that affect elementary-school aged kids, as well as adolescents, due to needing to adopt a strict adherence schedule for medications and other demands. McQueen added that it takes a long time and support to get the pediatric patients to a place where they can truly grow and be successful.

Social Worker Perspective

Charlie Thomas, social worker at the Banner-University Medical Center Phoenix, explained that every U.S. organ transplant center certified by the Centers for Medicare & Medicaid Services is required to have a state-licensed, master's level social worker. That way, he explained, every patient and family has access to a social worker, helping them navigate the process and outpatient posttransplant services. It begins a lifetime relationship with that patient and includes counseling, group work, and other services that are vital to their health and functioning.

Overview of Patient Challenges

Underscoring the realities related by the organ recipients and caregiver on the panel, Thomas presented a few of the major issues, including adjustment to chronic illness and ongoing treatment, relationship challenges, educational and vocational problems, crisis, chronic problem solving, as well as navigating difficult topics, such as end of life. Patients' and families' experiences are shaped most often by their insurance status, he added. Many have Medicaid or Medicare, making the government the largest payer of transplants in the country, but each insurance situation is different and often dictates how well patients do after transplantation. He shared findings from a 2001 study that, although QOL may improve for physical functioning, daily activities, and social functioning, various psychosocial problems confront the patient both before and after transplantation, with depression and anxiety being the most prevalent diagnoses (Engle, 2001). Other psychosocial problems included struggles with family roles and relationships, sexual dysfunction, return to work, adherence to a medical regimen, and anxiety about the possibility of organ rejection (Engle, 2001). Clinical outcomes were successful, Thomas said, yet mental and emotional health oftentimes suffered in the aftermath of the procedure. Caregivers are so important, noted Thomas, because after having access to so many medical experts and devices in the hospital, patients go home to a very different environment and need to manage their own care and treatment.

Difficulties Returning to Work

Thomas presented research on factors associated with returning to work. Paris et al. (1993) found that six factors were associated with return to work following a heart transplant:

- Physically able to work
- No loss of health insurance
- Longer length of time after transplant
- Education level higher than 12 years
- No loss of disability income
- Shorter length of disability before transplant

Thomas reported on another study that examined return to work after a heart transplant, which found associated factors to be age, length of disability before transplant, control over working conditions, and type of health insurance, including cost of medication (Meister et al., 1986). Of 47 patients, 32 percent returned to work, 25 percent retired, 7 percent were medically disabled, and 35 percent were "insurance disabled" (defined as fearing losing income and insurance by going back to work). Numbers from a study of kidney transplants were somewhat similar, with 57 percent of patients not working, but a high percentage (67 percent) with Medicaid reported that they were not working because they feared losing their health care benefits and not being able to afford immunosuppressive medications if they did go back to work (Markell et al., 1997).

Finally, Thomas shared recent results from a Swiss Transplant Consortium examining kidney, liver, heart, and lung transplant recipients: nearly 50 percent were employed by 12 months after transplantation, but the major predictor for this was pretransplant employment status (Vieux et al., 2019). He also commented that return to work was influenced by education level, depression levels 6 months after transplantation, and wait time in the employed group before transplantation—the longer unemployment was before transplantation, the longer it would take to be employed after.

DISCUSSION

McQueen began the discussion, asking others to highlight challenges recipients encounter when trying to manage their health, work, and family. Vlahos replied that the sheer volume of doctors' appointments, treatments, and medications really has a huge impact on daily life. She said that her transplant was not a cure for her CF; it gave her the gift of more time, but that time was not easily earned. Her transplant is at the forefront of all of her life decisions: where they live, where she works, what type of insurance they can get, or even where her husband works.

Regarding how the transplant has affected QOL, Edwards shared that her life has deteriorated. She ended up with other comorbidities, including bone diseases and early-stage colon cancer, and overall, it has affected her home life in a huge way, she said. While she can work somewhat, she has to carefully manage her schedule to ensure she does not do too much. She also struggles with mental health since her rejection episode and has been seeing a therapist. Keefer added that transplants come with many challenges before, during, and after the surgery. She also stressed the importance of the mental aspect and that it has not been emphasized enough in the field, and she advocated for more mental and emotional support for recipients. In response to other challenges navigating the system, Hoyt-Trapp highlighted the high levels of frustration and difficulty in trying to get services due to endless phone calls and paperwork. She said that while the initial recovery is coordinated through home health services, people have no centralized system available for different types of support or care after that. Making it even more difficult, she added, is that each state often has its own system, so things are not standardized. This is an issue for many patients who have to travel, or move, to other locations to obtain transplant services at specialized centers, which was also pointed out by Andrea DiMartini, professor of psychiatry and surgery at the University of Pittsburgh Medical Center in her presentation (see Chapter 3).

Montgomery asked about the most difficult period following the transplant procedure, and McQueen commented that the transplant itself is similar to a short sprint, but the posttransplant experience is a long-distance run. Her son had a feeding pump for 3 years and therapists for 4 years. While he is doing well now and in school, she recalled the first few years as very difficult. Vlahos added that recovery ebbs and flows. For her, the initial period was an incredible gift of being able to breathe on her own again. But several months later, she started suffering more severely from medication side effects, needed more surgeries, and depended on intravenous nutrition. In a final point, Montgomery noted the struggle is just getting started at 1 year after transplantation, but that is often where patients really start to feel a sudden void in services and support. He explained that transplant centers are held accountable for metrics up until 1 year, such as rates of patient and graft survival, for the purposes of financing and reimbursement. Because of this emphasis, he said, that is where the health care financing flows, leaving less support for the longer-term recovery.

3

Organ Transplantation and Disability in Adults

Many speakers described organ transplantation as a complex, lifesaving treatment that begins prior to the transplant and continues with many transitions and recovery periods in the months and years following. This chapter begins with summaries of Session 1 presentations and discussion, which addressed the clinical conditions that are associated with transplantation in adults and the consequences for health and function. Following those clinical overviews are summaries of Session 5A presentations and discussion in which speakers focused on physical, cognitive, and psychosocial functioning in adults after organ transplantation.

CLINICAL CONDITIONS AND CONSEQUENCES FOR HEALTH AND FUNCTION

In the first session, speakers discussed the most common types of solid organ transplants in adults—kidney, liver, lung, and heart—highlighting the causes of the end-stage organ disease, methods for estimating post-transplant survival, and statistics on survival and recovery outcomes across various patient groups. In addition, the presentations and panel discussion explored various factors that are associated with survival, recovery, and functioning in these transplant patients.

Kidney Transplantation

Dorry Segev, professor of surgery and epidemiology and associate vice chair of the Department of Surgery at Johns Hopkins University (JHU), discussed the prevalence of CKD and ESRD. CKD is the most common form of solid organ disease, affecting 37 million U.S. adults, 9 in 10 of whom may be unaware of it (CDC, 2021). All patients on the transplant waitlist are given an EPTS, a numerical score used to allocate donor kidneys. EPTS scores are designed to predict survival rates based on a variety of factors, including age, number of years on dialysis, presence of diabetes, and whether a candidate has had a prior solid organ transplant. Data published by the OPTN from deceased donor adult kidney transplants in 2008–2018 show that patients with an EPTS score of 0–20 percent had a 90 percent survival rate at 10 years after transplantation, whereas those with a score of 81–100 percent had only a 40 percent survival rate (OPTN, 2020a).

Donor factors are also important in evaluating transplant outcomes, as the quality of the donor kidney also largely impacts survival rates, Segev said. Donors are evaluated based on the kidney donor risk index (KDRI) and the kidney donor profile index (KDPI); KDRI values are calculated to determine the KDPI. Donor characteristics used to calculate the KDRI are age, height, weight, ethnicity, history of hypertension or diabetes, cause of death, serum creatinine, HCV status, and donation after circulatory death status. Similar to EPTS scores, the KDPI is also measured on a scale of 0–100 percent, where lower percentages indicate better graft survival rates. Data from 2008 to 2018 show that patients receiving a kidney with a KDPI of 0–20 percent had a graft survival of 60 percent at 10 years after transplantation, whereas those receiving a kidney with a KDPI of 86–100 percent had a 10-year graft survival of only 30 percent (OPTN, 2020b). As discussed by Mulligan, organs of all types are in short supply, including kidneys. Segev explained that the overall discard rate of kidneys due to poor KDPI is about 30 percent, whereas 70 percent of kidneys with high KDPI are deemed unfit for transplant (Bae et al., 2016).

Another factor strongly impacting kidney transplant survival rates is frailty, Segev said. The American Society of Transplantation has not set an upper age limit for transplant consideration, so patients with CKD at any age can be evaluated. However, Segev noted, frailty, disability, or dependence are associated with poor outcomes. Frail patients are 40 percent less likely to be added to the waiting list, and those who do make it onto the list are 32 percent less likely to ever receive a transplant and 1.7 times more likely to die waiting for a kidney (Haugen et al., 2019). Poor outcomes associated with frailty also include increased risk of mortality and early hospital readmission, increased risk of delayed graft function, and higher incidence of delirium (Garonzik-Wang et al., 2012; Haugen et al., 2018; McAdams-DeMarco et al., 2013a,b).

Segev discussed contraindications that may exclude eligibility for transplant. For example, absolute contraindications include active malignancy, acute infection, or vasculitis. Relative contraindications are cardiopulmonary disease, vascular disease, or uncontrolled psychiatric disorders. Other medical contraindications include bone disease, diabetes, hypertension, or anemia. However, Segev noted, all contraindications are evaluated case by case. When investigating cause of death after transplant, many of these contraindications are often present. Segev explained that 30–40 percent of deaths in kidney transplants are due to cardiovascular disorders, such as hypertension and diabetes, while 20–30 percent are due to infections, and an additional 20–30 percent are due to malignancy.[1] Segev concluded by highlighting that the heterogeneous nature of CKD patients leads to a variety of outcomes. Factors such as patient EPTS scores, donor KDPI scores, frailty, and medical contraindications all contribute to whether a kidney transplant will be successful.

Liver Transplantation

Shari Rogal, transplant hepatologist at the Pittsburgh Veterans Affairs Center for Health Equity Research and Promotion and assistant professor of medicine and transplant surgery at the University of Pittsburgh, began by sharing statistics about the prevalence of liver disease among U.S. adults. It is the 12th leading cause of death, and hepatocellular carcinoma, commonly known as "liver cancer," is the fastest growing cause of cancer death (Siegel et al., 2018). Consequently, she noted, the number of liver transplants per year is increasing and the patient population is older and sicker. Rogal shared data from the Scientific Registry of Transplant Recipients (SRTR) showing that in 2010, 11 percent of liver transplant recipients were over the age of 65, but that number doubled to 22 percent in 2020 (SRTR, 2018). She added that OPTN data show trends indicating survival rates can be predicted based on a patient's MELD score at the time of transplant: lower scores are predictive of a better chance of survival. Patients with a MELD

---

[1] Data courtesy of Dan Brennan, Johns Hopkins Medicine.

score below 15 at time of transplant have a 5-year survival rate of 84 percent, whereas patients with a score over 35 have a 5-year survival rate of about 74 percent (Kwong et al., 2020). As the population of liver transplant patients is aging, data also show that survival rates depend on age at transplant, she said. Data from Kwong et al. (2020) show that patients over 65 have a 5-year survival rate of 73 percent, whereas the 18–34 and 35–49 age groups both have a 5-year survival rate of 84 percent.

As the population makeup of liver transplant patients is changing, the causes of liver disease, or etiology, are changing as well. While 2.4 million people have liver disease associated with HCV, this number is decreasing (CDC, 2020b; Wong and Singal, 2020). Rogal explained that as HCV has become curable, those with HCV on the transplant waitlist are decreasing, while those on the list due to both alcohol use disorder and nonalcoholic steatohepatitis are nearly double the rate of HCV patients (Wong and Singal, 2020). Etiology is also a good indication of graft survival; patients with hepatocellular carcinoma have the poorest transplant outcomes, and those with HCV or cholesterol disease have significantly higher survival rates (Kwong et al., 2018). However, Rogal noted, the statistics are not all bad, citing a study that showed liver transplant survival rates remain extremely high, with 86 percent still alive at 1 year after transplantation and 72 percent at 5 years after transplantation (Kwong et al., 2018). The study also showed that the number of living donor transplants is increasing. While these are still a small percentage of total liver donations, Rogal explained that because donated livers are allocated based on disease severity and the sickest patients typically receive deceased donors' livers, the increase in living donors may indicate that more patients are receiving livers before extensive disease progression.

While survival rates for liver transplants are high, functional status remains relatively low 1 year after transplantation. Rogal shared that many patients report increases in physical distress, and more than half report limitations in the kind and amount of work they are able to do. Additionally, one in three patients is prevented from returning to work or school. A 12-year follow-up study showed many patients had no functional improvement at all (Ruppert et al., 2010). Rogal noted that while transplants may cure conditions such as liver cancer or metabolic diseases, they will not cure many underlying problems, whether they be physical, mental, or personal. Conditions such as diabetes, chronic pain, substance abuse disorder, depression, or financial problems are all obstacles that will remain after transplantation, and she added that some of these persistent problems, such as depression or chronic pain, may play a role in survival. Rogal noted that patients who have a history of depression have lower survival rates, and those who have been prescribed opioids for chronic pain are also less likely to have positive transplant outcomes. Approximately 80 percent of cirrhosis patients report experiencing chronic pain, and half of those are prescribed opioids for pain management (Rogal et al., 2015). Additionally, evidence suggests that higher doses of opioids at the time of transplant are associated with decreased survival rates (Randall et al., 2017).

Finally, Rogal ended by emphasizing that every patient is different. Despite many ways to predict survival rates, such as MELD score, age, and etiology (strong indicators of positive outcomes), patients have many physical, mental, and personal reasons that could lead them to need a liver transplant, such as substance abuse disorders or diabetes, that are not cured solely by transplanting the organ. She pointed out that as the prevalence of liver disease continues to rise in the United States, the number of patients presenting with more severe disease at the time of transplant, coupled with high survival rates, is leading to more people experiencing disability and decreased functional status after transplantation.

Lung Transplantation

Lung transplants in the United States are also rapidly increasing. In 2019, a record number of candidates were added to the waitlist, and the number of transplants performed continues to grow each year (Valapour et al., 2021). Erika Lease, transplant pulmonologist at the University of Washington, explained that the number of lung transplants in the United States is growing, particularly the number of patients undergoing a double lung transplant. Data from the SRTR show that lung transplants have nearly doubled in the past decade, from 1,500 in 2008 to almost 3,000 in 2019 (Valapour et al., 2021). While the majority of recipients are age 50–64, the number of patients over 65 is growing.

Lease explained that lung transplant patients generally belong to one of four major disease categories: chronic obstructive pulmonary disease (COPD), pulmonary fibrosis, CF, or pulmonary hypertension. COPD, a slow and progressive disease commonly attributed to smoking, is one of the most common forms of lung disease for which lung transplantation may be indicated; because of the slow nature of the disease, many patients are over the age of 60 and account for a large proportion of elder recipients (Chambers et al., 2019; Devine, 2008). Pulmonary fibrosis, however, is a common reason for lung transplant in older patients as well; patients generally have rapidly progressing disease and are typically transplanted within a few years of diagnosis. Pulmonary hypertension is another form of lung disease; blood vessels in the lungs become narrowed and can often lead to heart failure. Finally, the small portion of younger transplant recipients often suffers from CF, a lifelong genetic disease that leads to accumulating lung clogging and damage. Lease explained that these patients have the best survival rates, at almost 10 years, likely due to younger age at the time of transplant and lack of comorbidities.

Despite strides in the field of surgical techniques and posttransplant care, lung transplant long-term survival rates have not changed much in recent years. Lease explained that 10–15 percent of recipients will not survive the first year after transplantation and just under 50 percent will survive to 7 years. Since 1992, the median survival rate has only increased from 4.7 to 6.7 years (Chambers et al., 2019). Survival rates do differ depending on diagnosis and presence of comorbidities. While the median survival rate for CF patients, 9.9 years, is likely due to younger age at transplant, pulmonary fibrosis and COPD patients have the worst survival rates at 5.2 and 6 years, respectively. Lease explained these are likely due to older age at the time of transplant and smoking-related comorbidities in COPD patients (Chambers et al., 2019). Lease cited a variety of posttransplant complications that can lead to lower survival rates, such as recovering from a major thoracic surgery and pretransplant lung disease, adjusting to immunosuppressive medications, or chronic lung allograft dysfunction (CLAD), a progressive loss of lung function for which there is no effective treatment. Early transplant complications may arise, such as infection, which is the most common cause of death in the first year after transplant, or acute rejection. Patients are also at risk of later complications, many stemming from complications from the immunosuppressive medications, which can cause patients to develop comorbidities, including hypertension, diabetes, and even cancer. Lease indicated that long-term medication use can also lead to kidney damage; some patients may even require a kidney transplant. However, the biggest issue in later complications is CLAD, which Lease described as the greatest contributor to morbidity and mortality after the first year following transplant and showed that 43 percent of patients will have reported some kind of lung function decline by 5 years after transplantation (Valapour et al., 2021).

Lease concluded by emphasizing that the field of lung transplantation is constantly evolving, and survival is slowly improving. Survival rates can vary greatly depending on etiology, age, and comorbidities, but despite increasing survival rates, patients have to navigate a new set of challenges, including changes in QOL, functional status, and comorbidities that often result in the need for frequent medical care.

Heart Transplantation

One in four deaths in the United States is attributed to heart disease, claiming the lives of more than 650,000 Americans annually (CDC, 2020a; Virani et al., 2020). Hannah Valantine, professor of medicine at Stanford University, began by outlining the numerous indications that may warrant a heart transplant, such as refractory cardiogenic shock, recurring left ventricular arrhythmias, and end-stage congenital heart failure (Alraies and Eckman, 2014). In essence, these patients have extensive disease that has been unresponsive to multiple therapies, are unable to carry out everyday activities, and may even require assistive devices, such as an inter-aortic balloon pump. However, more than 80 percent of heart transplants are due to just two common conditions: ischemic cardiomyopathy and nonischemic cardiomyopathy. The former, commonly known as "coronary artery disease," has been responsible for 32.4 percent of heart transplants over the past decade; the latter, or heart failure without significant blockages to the coronary arteries, resulted in just over 50 percent of transplants (Khush et al., 2019). Valantine also noted that the number of patients bridged with mechanical support, or requiring mechanical circulatory assistive devices before transplant, is increasing. While only one-quarter of patients required a bridge to transplant in 2005, more than half did in 2017 (Khush et al., 2019). She explained that these patients requiring mechanical assistance are less likely to be able to fully rehabilitate and regain maximum function after transplantation.

As with all solid organ diseases, survival rates are largely dependent on etiology. Risk factors for mortality at both 1 year and 5 years after transplantation are similar, said Valantine, and include recipient age, body mass index, and kidney function as measured by creatinine levels. Survival risk factors also depend on the health of the donor, including age, cigarette use history, and donor–recipient predicted heart mass match (donor and recipient must be similar in weight) (Khush et al., 2019). Kidney function before transplantation is also particularly important due to the need for immunosuppressive medications after transplantation. Similar to lung transplant patients, she explained, heart transplant patients require many medications that put them at increased risk of kidney failure; 6.7 percent have severe renal dysfunction 1 year after transplantation and 15.7 percent 5 years after transplantation (Khush et al., 2019). Despite all of the necessary medications heart transplant recipients require, some will still experience rejection. Those who do, defined as having at least one acute rejection episode treated by an anti-rejection agent or being hospitalized for rejection, still equal 12 percent (Khush et al., 2019). Valantine explained that rejection is often treated with high-dose corticosteroids and other drugs that can put patients at risk for infection and require long periods of rehospitalization.

Despite the risk of complications, survival rates for heart transplant recipients are encouraging. Overall survival 1 year after transplantation is 91 percent, and it is 75 percent at 5 years, translating to median overall survival rates of 11.4 years for men and 12.2 years for women (Khush et al., 2019). Functional status and QOL after transplantation are also promising, Valantine added. She explained that 75 percent of patients report being able to carry out normal activity and 39 percent have returned to work 5 years after transplantation (Khush et al., 2019).

Valantine also discussed the three most common causes of death: malignancy, graft failure resulting in heart failure usually attributed to rejection, and cardiac allograft vasculopathy, a progressive blockage of the coronary arteries to the graft; she indicated that data from 1995 to 2018 show these three causes were responsible for 19.6 percent, 24.4 percent, and 12.4 percent of deaths, respectively. Valantine was optimistic about the median survival rate for heart transplant recipients being 11.6 years, and that as many as three in four are able to maintain good QOL and functional status. However, she added, a small percentage still battle disabling rejection and infection.

DISCUSSION

Paul Kimmel, program director at the Division of Kidney, Urologic, and Hematologic Diseases at the National Institute of Diabetes and Digestive and Kidney Diseases, moderated a discussion with the speakers from the first session. Reflecting on the challenges of returning to work, each speaker underscored that transplantation is only a treatment, not a cure. Moreover, recovery is extensive and a positive outcome is not always guaranteed, they cautioned. When thinking about posttransplant outcomes and disability, Kimmel asked why patients may enjoy good QOL but remain unable to return to work. Several experts agreed that a variety of factors are responsible for this disparity, such as the aging population of transplant recipients, mental health issues, and lack of employee protections. The lack of mental health care and poor social determinants of health in the United States also prevent many patients from returning to work, not because they are physically disabled but because they are not receiving adequate mental health and other psychosocial supports, as many workshop speakers pointed out. Underscoring this point, Segev implored clinicians to ask about emotional well-being rather than only focusing on physical health. He stressed the need for increased funding for mental health studies, while making the point that if only physical determinants of health, such as immunology and tissue engineering, are studied, that is all that will be known. Rogal also noted that patients who struggle with mental illness often turn to substance abuse, particularly alcohol and tobacco, which can also affect physical recovery and lead to poor outcomes. Finally, many patients do not return to work because of a lack of employee protections. Posttransplant care requires rigorous follow-up appointments that require time away from work. Purnell noted that hourly workers do not have the type of protections that salaried workers may have, such as the ability to take time off for these appointments. Many patients fear losing their disability benefits if they return to work, and hourly workers will not be paid while they take time off to attend medical appointments, leaving them without disability benefits or a paycheck. She added that labor laws and leave policies need to be examined and expanded to protect recipients from the fear of losing their jobs or benefits. Additionally, some may not be able to return to work due to unsafe working conditions given their new vulnerabilities. The fear of respiratory viruses or infection leaves many patients unable to return. Lease noted that many lung transplant recipients have experienced chronic allograft dysfunction after being exposed to respiratory viruses at work.

Kimmel posed a question about gaps in the available data, as transplant registries often lack functional data. David Mulligan responded that tracking long-term patient data lies largely on the shoulders of the transplant center and he suggested that patient self-reporting may lessen the burden. Furthermore, patients may relocate to posttransplant and transition care elsewhere rather than continuing care at their original transplant center. Several speakers identified a need to use new technology to report data, particularly in a way that makes it easy for patients to self-report data. Valantine also pointed out there are data gaps related to the social determinants of health, echoing Segev's previous comments by emphasizing "what gets measured gets done." Data on race, wealth, sex, and mental health are lacking because they are not always being measured, she argued. This again highlights the need to focus more on the "soft sciences," not only when treating patients but also while collecting data.

ASSESSING PHYSICAL, COGNITIVE, AND PSYCHOSOCIAL FUNCTION IN ADULTS AFTER ORGAN TRANSPLANTATION

As many speakers noted, the transplant journey does not end once the procedure is completed. Transplantation recovery is complex and thus answering questions regarding returning to work depend on many different factors. In Session 5A regarding adult physical, cognitive, and psychosocial functioning after transplantation, speakers described methods of assessing patient functioning and presented research findings on short- and long-term effects of transplantation on functioning and QOL. A panel discussion further explored the topic of impairments that can lead to disability following an organ transplant.

Physical Functioning

In order to talk about physical functioning after transplantation, a discussion about what happens to the body before transplant is necessary, said Jignesh Patel, medical director at Cedars-Sinai Medical Center. Due to end-stage organ disease, many patients end up with a physiologic state that results in significant disability. Patel defined "frailty" as a state of increased vulnerability to physiologic stress—distinct from aging, comorbidity, or disability—and noted the difficulty in quantifying frailty due to the lack of a gold standard assessment tool. Frailty is a common problem in organ transplants, he said, because of the nature of end-stage organ disease, and it manifests as decline in physical, psychosocial, and cognitive function. Patel indicated that the "Fried Criteria"[2] is the most extensively validated current tool and presented several studies that demonstrated that frail kidney transplant patients are at increased risk of poor outcomes. He noted that frailty is associated with more than 50 percent odds of a 2-week or longer length of hospital stay, almost twice the risk of delayed graft function, and more than twice the risk of mortality (Garonzik-Wang et al., 2012; McAdams-DeMarco et al., 2015, 2017). Looking closer at mortality associated with

---

[2] Fried's frailty model consists of five criteria—weight loss, exhaustion, low physical activity, slowness, and weakness—that are used for identifying frail older adults (Fried et al., 2001).

frailty after transplant across various organs, he emphasized that regardless of the organ type, being classified as frail prior to the transplantation nearly doubles the risk of mortality. The challenge, Patel continued, is transitioning a patient who has end-stage organ disease into a physically functioning state after transplantation. At an American Society of Transplantation conference convened on frailty, participants developed several concepts identifying it as common in patients (Kobashigawa et al., 2019). Patel explained that the conference noted that frailty affects mortality on the waitlist and in the posttransplant period. Participants discussed optimal methods to measure frailty, but these are yet to be determined or agreed upon. Patel also noted that interventions to reverse frailty are shown to vary among organ groups but so far appear promising. He summarized what happens in frailty and noted that the components include a range of factors across body systems, genetics, and the environment (see Figure 3-1). Age is certainly an important component, he acknowledged, as the greatest increase in demand for transplantation is seen by those above age 65, regardless of organ.

To address the issue of pretransplant frailty, Patel noted that attempts at prehabilitation have been made to see if patients can get stronger before the procedure, but these have shown limited efficacy. The most

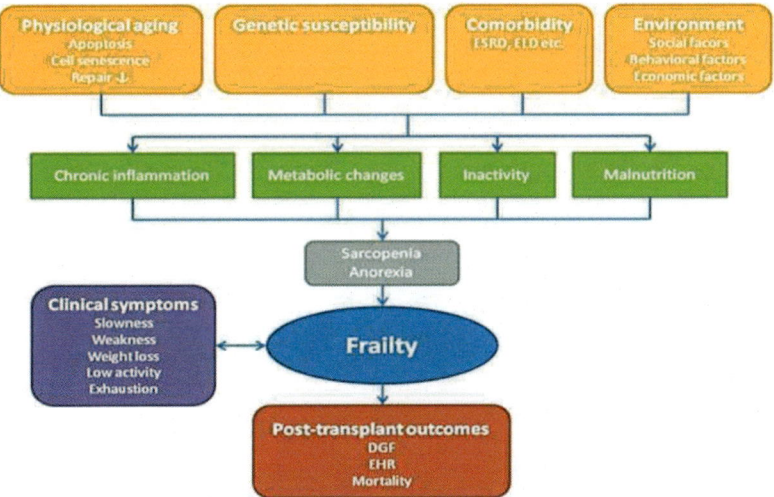

FIGURE 3-1 Summary of contributing factors leading to frailty.
NOTE: DGF = delayed graft function; EHR = early hospital readmission; ELD = end-stage liver disease; ESRD = end-stage renal disease.
SOURCES: Jignesh Patel presentation, March 23, 2021; Exterkate et al., 2016.

common intervention was exercise, but it has a large range in dropout rates—5–50 percent. Overall, exercise improved physical function, but the gains were modest compared to baseline level of impairment. Patel also described a clinical trial conducted by Kobashigawa et al. (1999), which measured exercise rehabilitation after heart transplant. Certain biomarkers improved following the intervention, he said, and other studies have shown that cardiac rehabilitation after a heart transplant was associated with significant decline in rehospitalization rates (Bachman et al., 2018). Similarly, in lung transplantation, a supervised exercise training intervention in the first 3 months after transplant was associated with increased functional capacity—at 3 months and even 1 year afterward (Langer, 2015). In longer-term studies, nearly half of patients reported no functional disability—but those who did cited more clinical symptoms, depression, and other comorbidities. They were more often older, female, less educated, and unemployed (Grady et al., 2007).

Measuring physical functioning continues to be a challenge, but new technology is becoming more commonly used and integrated into monitoring. Patel highlighted activity trackers or wearable devices that offer feedback to adjust activity in near real time—something that looks promising but is still being evaluated, he added. Essentially, physical functioning after an organ transplant is highly dependent on pretransplant state. Frailty is very common, said Patel, and despite some efforts to address frailty prior to transplant, most efforts thus far have focused on the posttransplant phase.

Cognitive Functioning

Aditi Gupta, associate professor of medicine at the University of Kansas Medical Center, opened by sharing that an inspiration for her research career was a patient who mentioned the brain fog they suffered from disappeared following a transplant. Gupta pointed out that cognitive impairment is common; she shared a study of patients on dialysis that found up to 87 percent have some form of cognitive impairment, with just 13 percent having normal cognitive function (Murray et al., 2006). Cognitive impairment influences kidney transplant eligibility, Gupta noted. She shared findings from her study that showed subclinical cognitive impairment is associated with a lower likelihood of being listed for a kidney transplant and a longer time getting to transplant (Gupta et al., 2019). Gupta explained that kidney transplant recipients have a high prevalence of cognitive impairment, regardless of age. However, despite this knowledge becoming more widely available, she said it is not currently the standard of care to measure cognition in pretransplant or posttransplant care, and most centers do not even have the resources to do so or screen for cognitive impairment.

Gupta stated that although many clinicians feel that they could reliably detect some type of cognitive impairment in their patients, this may not be the case. Gupta described a study showing that the clinicians' perceptions of cognitive impairment in patients matched the "measured" cognition scores (using a standardized assessment tool) only about half the time (Gupta et al., 2018). The exact etiology of cognitive impairment is multifactorial but unknown, she explained. Ongoing studies are examining the possible role of anti-rejection medications, such as calcineurin inhibitors, which are potent vasoconstrictors and hypothesized to potentially decrease cerebral blood flow and affect cognition. Focusing more on the connection between CKD and brain abnormalities, Gupta said that it is well established, and the specific brain abnormalities that CKD causes are associated with cognitive impairments also seen in non-CKD populations. To understand these connections better, she shared a study that examined brain magnetic resonance imaging (MRI) before, 3 months after, and 12 months after transplant and found that where blood flow in the brain was higher before transplantation, it decreased after transplant—even below the original baseline (Lepping et al., 2021).

Looking more broadly, Gupta discussed several longitudinal studies assessing change in cognition from pre- to post-kidney transplant. Not a lot of data are available, and research is ongoing, she said, but overall, all studies give the same message—certain domains of cognition do improve after transplantation, but overall cognition does not totally normalize. She highlighted one study that demonstrated improved logical memory, but no improvements in other areas of cognition after kidney transplant (Gupta et al., 2017). Gupta noted that preliminary data from cognition analysis studies correlated with brain changes detected in MRIs. She said short screening tests are not sensitive enough to appreciate the change in cognition, and current information is insufficient about which domains and which areas of the brain improve. Gupta explained that the current thinking is most of the chronic brain damage being measured happened before the transplant and is not completely reversible, but studies are still ongoing. Overall, she concluded that cognitive impairment is highly prevalent among transplant recipients but the field still needs better ways to assess cognition. She pointed out that mechanisms for underlying deficits in cognitive impairment vary among different solid organs, so findings from one organ to another should not be extrapolated. Finally, there are not currently enough data to be able to predict posttransplant cognition scores based on pretesting.

Psychosocial and Emotional Functioning

Transplantation is not merely the singular event related to the surgery; it is a journey that begins before that, with discrete transition and recovery periods, said Andrea DiMartini, professor of psychiatry and surgery at the University of Pittsburgh. DiMartini explained that after patients are put on the waitlist, while waiting for a donated organ to become available, they may become sicker, with acute health crises and deteriorating physical health. Many patients maintain hope but still recognize the possibility that a transplant might not occur, which can result in great emotional stress. When patients receive an organ, there is an initial posttransplant period where they are elated to have received this second chance but then realize there is a lot of physical recovery to be achieved, which can be really discouraging, DiMartini said. They also may face the constant worry of organ rejection or rehospitalization and the stress of adjusting to powerful daily immunosuppressive medications. As they begin to adapt to their new lives and responsibilities, they also try to resume their previous life and may consider going back to work, creating a lot of potential stressors. The long-term maintenance phase, she added, may include chronic rejection, recurrent organ disease, or even a need for a second transplant, so stress may continue even many years later.

QOL is an important metric of physical and mental well-being, said DiMartini. Virtually all studies show that transplant recipients show some improvement in QOL, but the level is more comparable to others with chronic disease as compared to that of healthy people. In terms of mental well-being, DiMartini noted that the first year following transplant has shown mood and anxiety disorders, ranging from 20 percent for kidney recipients to as high as 60 percent for heart recipients (DiMartini et al., 2008). Anxiety specifically appears to be prominent in lung recipients, and posttraumatic stress disorder (PTSD) can sometimes develop from the transplant experience. PTSD may cause avoidance of future appointments because of the anxiety that it triggers. The rates of onset of mental health disorders appear to follow a certain pattern after transplantation. She shared findings from Dew et al. (2001) that examined heart transplant recipients and found their first year was particularly stressful, which is expected, she said. Although the prevalence of depressive or anxiety disorders declined over subsequent years, she noted that it then plateaued and began to increase again around 10 years after transplantation, perhaps at the time where patients begin to experience additional health problems. Certain mental health disorders are linked to poor medical outcomes, DiMartini stated. Depression is a primary example—it is associated with unhealthy physiologic changes, such as inflammation, lethargy, fatigue, poor sleep, and poor appetite. A meta-analysis showed that among transplant recipients across all organ types, those who had a pre- or posttransplant history of depression had significantly poorer survival rates and increased graft loss (Dew et al., 2015). She also highlighted a possible correlation in liver recipients between posttransplant depression and unemployment but noted that the temporal relationship between this linkage was unknown, and more research is still needed to determine its direction (Newton, 2003).

Strategies to Improve Mental Health Outcomes and Support Return to Work

DiMartini began by stating that clinical strategies that consider patients' lives before transplant and that prepare them for transplantation during the pretransplant phase can help improve posttransplant outcomes. In addition to ensuring patients have sufficient social support, she emphasized the need to prepare patients for realistic expectations regarding physical outcomes and long-term functioning, with varying plans on returning to work, depending on each individual. She shared findings from Rogal et al. (2013) illustrating the importance of this early identification and treatment of mental health issues, where researchers found liver recipients who were given adequate antidepressant therapy had better survival rates than those with depression who were untreated. It appeared that adequate treatment may reduce mortality risk conferred by depression, she explained. DiMartini offered some interventions that clinicians can suggest to assist recipients in their quest to return to work (see Box 3-1).

In summary, DiMartini said, placing the strongest efforts into the first year after transplantation, where stress and rates of mental health disorders are high, and focus on mental health and recovery may help to maximize long-term outcomes.

DISCUSSION

Erika Lease and Shari Rogal moderated a discussion with the Session 5A speakers on the various methods for assessing and improving physical and

> **BOX 3-1**
> **Interventions for Clinicians to Assist**
> **Recipients in Return to Work**
>
> - Thorough assessment of mental health, motivation, desire, and ability to return to work;
> - Formal neuropsychological testing and cognitive rehabilitation if indicated;
> - Physical rehabilitation can improve physical functioning through structured exercise training and/or physical rehabilitation;
> - For those returning to a prior job, emotional support may help in transition; and
> - Employment counseling, aptitude testing, and assistance with job placement.[a]
>
> ---
>
> [a] One observational study using a multipronged QOL intervention after kidney transplant, of which employment/vocational counseling was one component, found 86 percent of those employed prior to transplant returned to work by 6 months after transplantation (Chang et al., 2004).
> SOURCE: Andrea DiMartini presentation, March 23, 2021.

cognitive functioning in adult transplant recipients. Lease asked Patel how effective posttransplant interventions are for frailty and whether the improvements seen are sustainable. Patel responded that the data supporting interventions are strongest for heart transplants, where cardiac rehabilitation has been shown to significantly improve functional capacity, QOL, and cognition and translate into long-term benefits. Because of this, cardiac rehabilitation is now a routine part of care, but this is less so for other organs, where the evidence is less established. But Patel commented that the general changes resulting in frailty are common to all organ transplants, so presumably the improvements found from posttransplant cardiac rehabilitation would be applicable across other solid organs.

Lease asked Gupta whether patients can recognize cognitive impairment in themselves or if they must rely on a medical provider to identify and address it. Gupta said that the patients will generally feel it, likely sooner than a medical provider would notice, but it is subjective. She said the only way for providers to really identify cognitive decline is to conduct formal testing, which is less focused on an absolute score but instead something to watch over time to see how it changes. Once the presence of cognitive decline or impairment has been established, Gupta noted that the success of the intervention will depend on the mechanism of the issue, as some will be more reversible than others. For example, in kidney disease, reasons could be related to the disease directly, even before transplantation, or cognitive decline could be because of calcineurin inhibitors or other immunosuppressive agents that constrict blood flow, but she said it is unknown whether they affect cerebral flood flow. Additionally, cognitive decline could be related to the surgical process, she said; kidney transplant surgeries are typically shorter and easier on the body, compared to heart or lung transplants, which are longer and cause more hypotension and postoperative delirium.

Numerous barriers to recovery are also related to psychosocial and emotional function, which can make it difficult for patients to resume their lives. DiMartini noted that if patients are not being screened for mental health problems, then it is difficult to pick up on how they are doing. Unless transplant recipients are asked appropriate questions about how they are doing emotionally, she said, it is easy to overlook those who are experiencing significant depression or anxiety. Providing patients with appropriate mental health treatment so symptoms are in remission before the surgery is important, DiMartini said. But, she added, this can be challenging because many patients travel out of state for transplant care. Obtaining mental health care can be particularly problematic either because the provider is located in a different state, which can be difficult with telemedicine regulations, or the provider is separate from the transplant program, which can make it hard for some patients to maintain regular appointments.

Lease also asked about comorbidities that arise from posttransplant treatment and if some are more common or more limiting than others. Patel responded that most are directly related to immunosuppression medication effects. For example, diabetes becomes much more prevalent in this population, as well as high blood pressure and obesity. Together, these comorbidities can certainly affect QOL and functioning. Gupta agreed on the importance of rehabilitation programs in the early posttransplant phases but commented that many patients who receive organ transplants do not have access to them. She highlighted many studies that show patients do really well mentally and physically in active intervention programs after transplantation, but when they end, things tend to return to the way they were before the research study. Therefore, some kind of longer-term maintenance program is needed, she said. DiMartini added that depression is a significant comorbidity that can affect every area of life and functioning, including whether someone is taking recommended medications. She emphasized that inadequately treated depression in transplant patients can affect not only QOL but also survival. In one study, patients who were depressed were approximately 2.5 times more likely to die in subsequent posttransplant years as compared to patients who were not depressed (Rogal et al., 2013).

Impact of COVID-19 on Posttransplant Functioning

Lease asked all speakers whether they know what impact active COVID-19 infection has had on transplant recipients' posttransplant functional abilities, directly or indirectly. Gupta replied, noting the differences between "active COVID" and "long COVID," where patients suffer from fatigue and sometimes cognitive impairment for months afterward. Many questions remain about how these symptoms would intersect with posttransplant symptoms in a transplant recipient. Patel added that they do know mortality rates for transplants are very high at 20–25 percent for hospitalized patients. Emerging data show the vaccine may not be fully protective for transplant recipients (Boyarsky et al., 2021), which naturally is leading to anxiety for those who are feeling vulnerable. DiMartini also emphasized this point, calling attention to the anxiety and depression levels—even substance use relapse—by patients who are very concerned with getting infected and are afraid to leave the house. Lease agreed COVID-19 has significantly impacted early posttransplant management and care. She added that getting people access to physical functioning rehabilitation was extremely difficult with most of the programs closed during the previous year.

Final Thoughts on Changes to Improve Outcomes

In conclusion, Rogal asked each speaker to suggest changes to policies or other factors that could improve outcomes. DiMartini emphatically responded that insurance and access to care would be her focus areas, because she struggles to find mental health resources that are covered by insurance, no matter what location patients are in at the time. Patel agreed and added that access to physical rehabilitation in the early posttransplant phase is also critical. Investing in rehabilitation services is important, he said, because they can help reduce rehospitalization rates and comorbidities and improve survival and return-to-work rates.

4

Organ Transplantation and Disability in Children and Adolescents

While the majority of transplant patients are adults, hundreds of children undergo solid organ transplantation each year in the United States. Similar to Chapter 3, but addressing special concerns of children and adolescents, this chapter summarizes the presentations and discussions in Session 2 regarding the clinical conditions that are associated with the most common pediatric organ transplants and the consequences for health and function. This is followed by summaries of the Session 5B presentations and discussions in which speakers focused on physical, cognitive, and psychosocial functioning in children after organ transplantation, as well as the specific challenges that adolescents face.

CLINICAL CONDITIONS AND CONSEQUENCES FOR HEALTH AND FUNCTION

Session 2 speakers presented clinical overviews of liver and intestine, kidney, lung, and heart transplants in children and adolescents that highlighted the causes of the end-stage organ disease, methods for estimating posttransplant survival, and statistics on survival and recovery outcomes across various groups. In addition, the presentations and panel discussion explored various factors that are associated with survival, recovery, and functioning in these patients.

Liver and Intestine Transplantation

George V. Mazariegos, chief of pediatric transplantation at the University of Pittsburgh Medical Center Children's Hospital of Pittsburgh, began with an overview of liver and intestine transplantation in children, noting that the number of pediatric liver transplants is approximately five times more than the number of pediatric intestine transplants each year. He said that the number of pediatric liver transplants has been fairly stable over the past decade, whereas the number of intestinal transplants is decreasing—primarily because of hormonal therapy improvements and other medical advances in the treatment of gut diseases. He indicated that a key trend is the ability to do technical variant liver transplants,[1] which offers children an option that has reduced waitlist mortality, possibly eliminating it entirely. Retransplantation is fairly rare for liver recipients, he added, with just 10 percent needing one within 15 years. However, 15 percent of intestine recipients may require a retransplant within 5 years (Kwong et al., 2021). Mazariegos shared additional findings based on OPTN/SRTR data: more than 27,000 U.S. children are living with a functional allograft today, with liver and kidney transplants being the highest, compared to fewer heart recipients and significantly fewer intestine and lung recipients.

Before discussing the factors that can lead to liver or intestinal transplantation, Mazariegos reviewed a three-tiered hierarchy of outcome measures, a concept that can be applied to any chronic disease or therapy, allowing caregivers and families to understand the different tiers of care that can occur over the life cycle of a certain condition (Porter, 2010; see Figure 4-1). In the surgical transplant world, Mazariegos explained that patient outcome assessments most often address Tier 1, centering on survival. Tier 2 is focused on the process of recovery, the time it takes, and how well patients can return to healthy living. Tier 3 covers sustainability of health. This third tier asks whether the condition is successfully treated after transplantation, if disease recurs, and what long-term consequences of any therapy might be. If patients develop other diseases or need retransplantation, the cycle would start again.

To help understand how liver and intestine transplants may be similar or different, Mazariegos discussed what diseases lead to transplantation in children. For those requiring a liver transplant, the most common conditions are chronic liver disease and metabolic or genetic conditions, which together account for more than 50 percent of the indications for pediatric

---

[1] Technical variant techniques use a partial liver graft to replace the role of a whole organ.

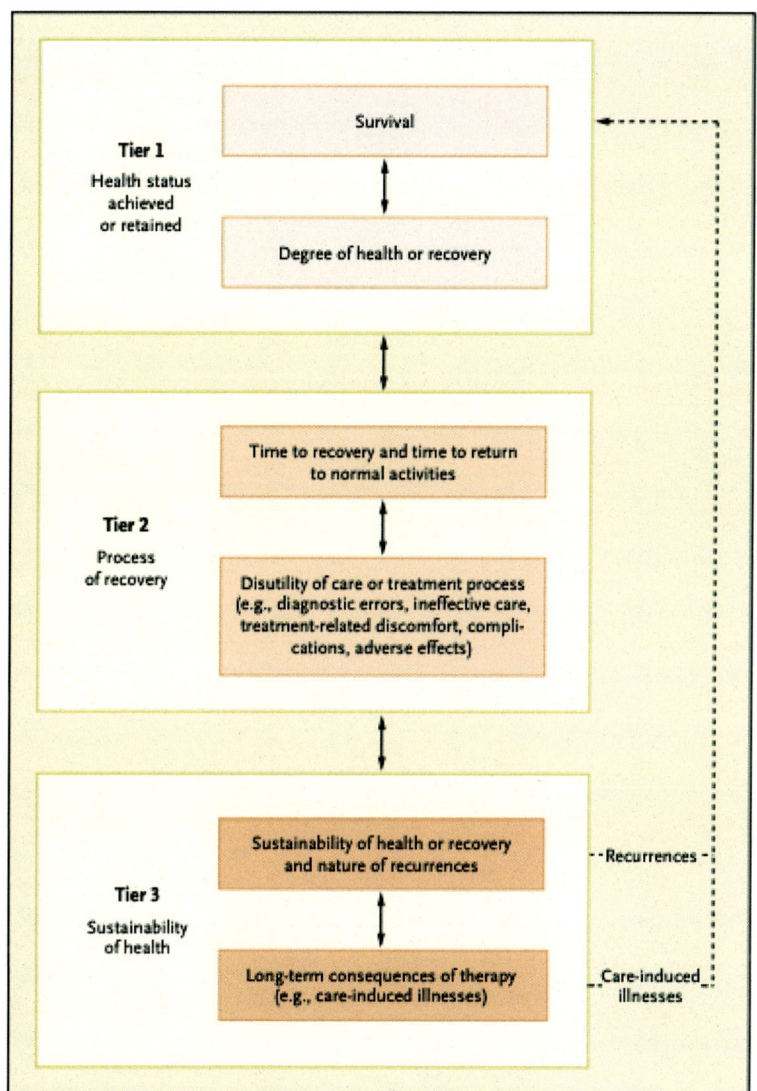

FIGURE 4-1 Hierarchy of outcome measures.
SOURCES: George Mazariegos presentation, March 22, 2021; Porter, 2010.

liver transplants in the United States (Squires et al., 2014). For those needing an intestine transplant, 70 percent of indications relate to loss of the intestine from surgical removal due to a condition such as necrotizing enterocolitis (Horslen et al., 2021). The other 30 percent are due to motility disorders, but systemic conditions leading to gut loss are generally rare (Horslen et al., 2021). In chronic liver disease, many of the associated comorbidities are attributable to malnutrition or liver failure and will improve following transplant. But in some children with metabolic disease, the ongoing systemic condition may not allow a complete return to normal even after transplantation, highlighting the ongoing systemic effect of the metabolic complications.

In terms of long-term outcomes, Mazariegos explained that liver transplant recipients fare significantly better than patients requiring intestine transplants. Only about 25 percent of liver recipients from deceased donors had graft failure after 10 years, compared to 40–60 percent of intestine recipients (Kwong et al., 2021). Most who received a liver transplant since 1989 still have their first allograft. Thinking specifically about liver and intestine transplants within the tiered outcome model (see Figure 4-1), he said the degree of recovery for liver transplant recipients is excellent, with good short- and long-term outcomes (see Figure 4-2). In comparison, pediatric intestine transplant patients have a more challenging survival and degree of recovery, shown in Figure 4-3. Survival is generally good compared to death from the significant morbidities of their disease, but only 40 percent of patients needing intestine transplantation have long-term survival.

In his concluding remarks, Mazariegos called for transitioning to a more holistic standard when viewing outcome metrics. He presented a study conducted by Ng et al. (2012) looking at liver transplants 10 years

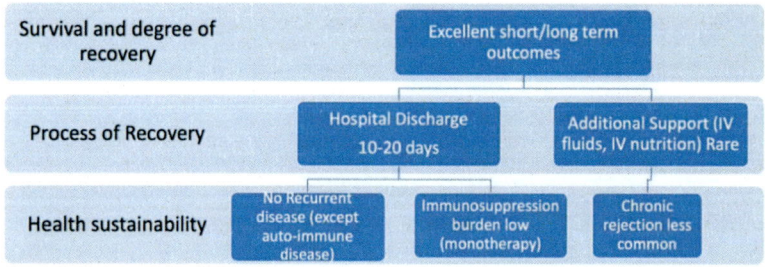

FIGURE 4-2 Pediatric liver transplantation across three tiers of outcomes.
NOTE: IV = intravenous.
SOURCE: George Mazariegos presentation, March 22, 2021.

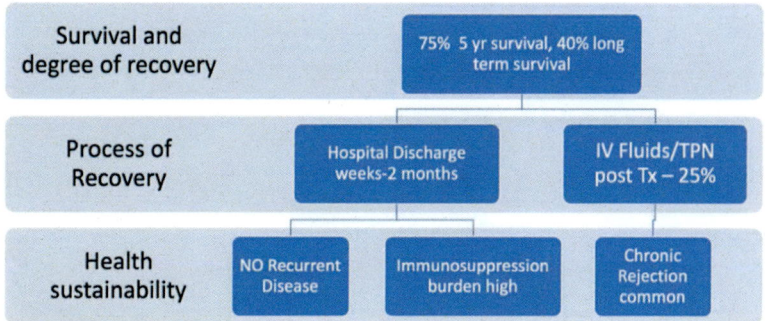

FIGURE 4-3 Pediatric intestine transplantation across three tiers of outcomes.
NOTE: IV = intravenous; TPN = total parenteral nutrition; Tx = treatment.
SOURCE: George Mazariegos presentation, March 22, 2021.

after transplantation, which examined how the liver was functioning and what extra hepatic measures of an ideal outcome were present, including QOL. While most of the 10-year survivors had achieved most of the measures, only about one-third achieved all 13 of them. Marzariegos stated he believes liver and intestine transplants are best evaluated through an outcomes hierarchy to identify the distinct challenges children face through the transplant journey, as their cycle of care is measured in decades compared to years for adults.

Kidney Transplantation

Maria E. Diaz-Gonzalez de Ferris, professor of pediatrics at the University of North Carolina at Chapel Hill, focused her presentation on kidney transplants in children and young adults. She first presented data from 2015 to 2018 showing the difference in causes of end-stage kidney disease by age. Children who are diagnosed young, especially less than 1 year old, she said, are more likely to have congenital abnormalities of the kidney and urinary tract. But in children diagnosed later, the causes are more likely to be glomerular disease or other conditions. She added that the incidence and prevalence of end-stage kidney disease in children have really remained stable in the United States. While adults typically have a 10-year survival rate of about 50 percent, children often fare much better, and have 10-year survival rates of 85–90 percent, an increase from the 70 percent range in the 1970s (Ferris et al., 2006).

Diaz-Gonzalez de Ferris explained what it means if a child has end-stage kidney disease. Pediatric patients can have comorbidities, just like adults, but also may experience cognitive impairment, learning abnormalities, mood disorders, gastrointestinal disturbances, and even dental abnormalities. She added that cardiovascular disease plays a significant role in a child's prognosis, and those who survive to their 30s and 40s may have the same cardiovascular risk as an 80-year-old. Diaz-Gonzalez de Ferris indicated that the mental and emotional burden on these pediatric patients adds another challenge, as they often have low levels of employment in adulthood, low self-esteem, and diminished health-related QOL. In addition, she said that adolescents and young adults with chronic of end-stage kidney disease are at great risk of nonadherence to medication regimens and provider follow-ups. She explained that it is difficult for them to self-manage their disease in part because typical individuals do not reach brain maturity until their mid-20s, and the cognitive effects of end-stage kidney disease may delay full maturity. Diaz-Gonzalez de Ferris presented on Gogtay et al. (2004), which measured brain activity in healthy controls compared to pediatric kidney disease patients and found that the latter had decreased activation in the parietal lobe and prefrontal regions of the brain. She said that these children may take longer to mature, and even at full maturity, they may not have formed all of their neural connections.

Once pediatric patients with chronic conditions, including those who have received a transplant, have transferred to adult-oriented care, Diaz-Gonzalez de Ferris said, they often do not have a great deal of knowledge about their diagnosis and medications, are often nonadherent, and may continue to be dependent on their parents. Diaz-Gonzalez de Ferris cautioned that when adolescent patients with chronic conditions are not prepared to self-manage their care as adults, they can experience adverse effects, including transplant rejection, death, graft loss, higher hemoglobin A1C scores in diabetics, and increased arthritis activity. Reporting findings from a study that measured transition readiness among adolescents and young adults (Zhong et al., 2018), she said that while many with chronic conditions succeed at mastering different parts of their condition along the way, it was not until they were in their 20s that they fully learned to self-manage their health. Thus, Diaz-Gonzalez de Ferris noted, programs that teach patients about health self-management and focus on this transition are important. She described research that found adolescents significantly preferred learning about their health conditions from their parents or provider, as compared to the Internet, other patients, or written information (Johnson et al., 2015). These preferences were associated with greater adherence to treatment protocols, self-efficacy, and transition readiness. See Adolescent Transitions to Adulthood After Transplantation below for additional information on this topic.

Lung Transplantation

Pediatric lung transplants are very rare, said Carol Conrad of Lucile Packard Children's Hospital, with only 37 pediatric lung transplant centers around the world, mostly in North America and Europe. At her center in California, they perform three to five pediatric lung transplants each year. She explained the wide range in causes of end-stage lung disease, differing by the age of the child. CF is the most common reason in older children and teenagers, with an average of 58 each year worldwide. Infants are commonly referred for pulmonary hypertension, which often develops secondary to a cardiovascular malformation. Other causes include interstitial lung diseases from genetic mutations or rheumatologic disorders, but these types of disorders require very few lung transplants annually. Conrad presented a survival curve comparing rates between children and adults, with median survival for adults being 8.3 years and children 9.1 years. However, she did note that survival has been improving since 2010 (Hayes et al., 2019). When breaking down the data for children into more discrete age groups, she explained that younger children have better outcomes compared to adolescents. This is in part due to adolescents' new sense of independence and poorer adherence to recovery treatments, Conrad said.

Conrad discussed how transplant centers estimate the level of impairment in a patient prior to transplantation through a combination of aerobic and mobility testing, muscle function, and assessment of physical activity level. However, many pediatric patients with lung diseases are unable to complete a 6-minute walking test because of their limited lung function, Conrad said. If their lungs are scarred or have limited blood flow, they are unable to increase their lung volume, leading to low oxygen levels. Conrad emphasized that optimal physical function and condition before lung transplantation contributes to better outcomes. She referenced studies in both pediatric and adult candidates that demonstrate that rehabilitation exercises before transplantation can lead to an improved exercise activity level and increase in the 6-minute walk distance (Castleberry et al., 2017). She said these gains are correlated with improved patient survival while on the lung transplant waiting list, fewer days on mechanical ventilation, and shorter stays in the ICU after transplantation for both children and adults. Posttransplant complications can decrease from exercise training and proper nutrition, but she stated it is still unknown whether these interventions affect longer-term survival, though the QOL implications are clear. No specific guidelines exist for determining the level of fitness for candidates, but many options are available. Conrad noted that many providers monitor patients with gross motor exercise tests, along with other tools such as developmental milestones, a pediatric multidimensional fatigue scale, or functional status estimates through the Lansky performance scale.[2] She presented data showing the functional status of surviving pediatric recipients at 1-, 2-, and 3-year follow-up visits from 2008 through 2017, as displayed in Figure 4-4. Conrad explained that by 3 years after transplantation, nearly 80 percent of recipients reported normal function, and another 10 percent were active but tired easily.

Conrad suggested pediatric lung transplant recipients would likely benefit from a directed treatment rehabilitation exercise program to achieve their best functionality and QOL. Given the limitations, she said, they focus on a better QOL rather than length of survival. Rehabilitation and physical therapy are important tools to help them achieve normal activities in their lives, including school, sports, and good physical, social, and mental health outcomes. Finally, she advocated for sharing and testing methodologies between transplant centers to better understand which interventions can best produce these outcomes to support their patients.

Heart Transplantation

Nine out of every 1,000 live births result in a child with congenital heart disease (CHD), stated Clifford Chin, director of Advanced Cardiomyopathy Services and medical director of Pediatric Heart Transplant at Cincinnati Children's Hospital Medical Center (AHA, 2021). Chin went on to say that one-third of those will require surgery early in their lives. CHD is one of the major reasons a child might need a transplant, in addition to cardiomyopathy, a condition where the heart cannot pump enough blood needed for the body. Eventually, dilated cardiomyopathies overcome CHD as the leading indication for transplantation among adolescents. While neurological complications can be quite common, Chin said it is difficult to discern whether cognitive neurologic defects exist prior to cardiac

---

[2] The Lansky performance scale measures QOL, including psychosocial and functional status, in children (Lansky et al., 1987).

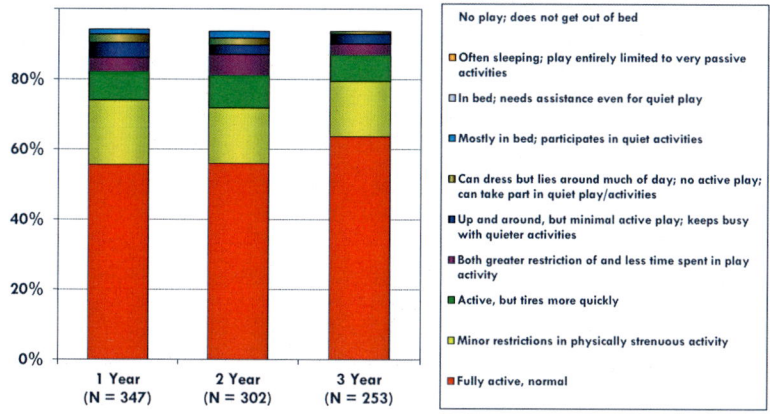

FIGURE 4-4 Functional status of surviving pediatric lung transplant recipients.
SOURCES: Carol Conrad presentation, March 22, 2021; International Society for Heart and Lung Transplantation (ISHLT) International Thoracic Organ Transplant (TTX) Registry.

surgery in infants. Nonetheless, infant patients are at highest risk for severe developmental delay, which has consequences for future employability, insurability, educational achievement, and physical activity. Worldwide, Chin highlighted that approximately 25 percent of pediatric heart transplants each year occur in infants (Dipchand et al., 2013); children between the ages of 1 and 10 make up approximately 35 percent. Each year, the United States has roughly 500 heart transplants in children, defined as receiving a new heart prior to reaching their 18th birthday.

Chin described QOL assessment tools, including the Pediatric QOL Inventory tool (PedsQL), which assesses five domains of health: physical, emotional, psychosocial, social, and school functioning. The health-related QOL Inventory focuses more specifically on the effects of illness and the impact that treatment may have on QOL. Generally, children with more severe cardiovascular disease experience poorer physical and psychosocial QOL. Chin reported that even after transplantation, heart recipients have lower health-related QOL compared to children who are healthy, have chronic conditions, or have CHD. Going into transplant, children of different age categories will present differently but are generally very ill and may require life support. Chin stated that older children and adolescents who have had multiple surgeries typically do not require hospitalization while waiting for a heart but are often not well enough to attend school. Similarly, cardiomyopathy patients considered for transplant are generally too fragile to attend school and are often hospitalized for months on intravenous medications. Some develop severe dysfunction of the heart, requiring mechanical support devices, which can lead to other health risks.

Describing what may happen after a heart transplant, Chin said that a clock begins that will count down until the patient passes away or requires a second transplant. Chin explained that the half-life[3] for pediatric patients to arrive at this point is approximately 20 years but varies depending on the age at transplant (Rossano et al., 2019). Chin indicated that infants have better overall survival outcomes as compared to teenagers. He said that if 100 infants received a transplant today, one would expect 50 of them to be alive with their first transplanted heart in 25 years. On the other hand, if 100 teenagers were transplanted today, 50 of them would be alive in only 14 years. Chin added that because of improvements in half-life during the past two decades, cardiac retransplantation in pediatric patients is uncommon. For those that do require transplantation, the half-life of the second transplant is shorter; it may be only 10 years.

Chin described a number of clinical consequences pediatric patients may experience after heart transplantation. He said many patients develop kidney disease and described risk factors for the development of kidney disease this include preexisting disease, effects of surgery and hospitalization, use of anti-rejection medications, and age at transplant. While the majority of children do not experience severe kidney disease at 10 years after transplantation, Chin said that 10–15 percent of the population will require some form of dialysis by 20 years. He mentioned cancer is a problem that affects a small number of transplant patients and that most of the cancers that do develop are thought to be due to immunosuppressive medications in combination with certain viruses, especially Epstein-Barr virus infection, that can lead to the development of lymphoma. Chin also reported on repeated posttransplant hospitalizations, saying that although they do decrease over time, even 5 years after transplantation, 30 percent of patients are readmitted due largely to rejection and infection (Rossano et al., 2019). In terms of function, 70 percent of children report being fully active after 3 years, with the majority of the remainder having some limitations on strenuous activity (Rossano et al., 2019).

---

[3] Half-life is the time required for a quantity to reduce to half of its initial value; in the context of transplantation, it refers to the time it takes for half of the grafts functioning at 1 year to subsequently fail.

Chin explained that it is possible to objectively measure exercise capacity and quantitate functional status. Compared to healthy children, pediatric transplant recipients have reduced exercise capacity, including lower peak oxygen consumption, higher resting heart rate, and lower peak heart rate. Cardiac rehabilitation programs and the significant benefits they can provide (increased in exercise capacity and muscle strength) are not widely available to children. Chin noted that compared to the 2,500 certified adult cardiac rehabilitation programs in the United States, there are just 10–15 certified pediatric programs. Currently, he said, pediatric heart transplant patients are set up to be deconditioned and less active, which leads to a weak foundation as they transition to adulthood.

Finally, cardiac transplantation is not a cure, Chin emphasized. While it is a lifesaving treatment, it creates a chronic health condition that depends on medications with adverse effects and limits to daily activities. Developmental delay and impaired cognitive function, the absence of pediatric resources to improve physical health, and inherent problems of transitioning from pediatric to adult programs are just a few of the barriers that hinder success for these patients.

ADOLESCENT TRANSITIONS TO ADULTHOOD AFTER TRANSPLANTATION

Transitioning to adult-oriented care is a challenging endeavor for many adolescent recipients. In Session 2, Nitika Gupta, professor of pediatrics at the Emory University School of Medicine, presented the current status of this transition, expanding on several points made earlier by Diaz-Gonzalez de Ferris. Four million young adults in the United States turn 18 each year, with 18–20 percent of them affected by chronic health conditions (Goodman et al., 2011). This translates to around 750,000 patients with special needs transitioning from pediatric to adult health care every year, she said, and less than half receive adequate support and services (Goodman et al., 2011; McManus et al., 2013; Rosen et al., 2003). Evidence suggests this transition is associated with adverse health outcomes (Toomey et al., 2013). Gupta stated that, based on OPTN data, children make up approximately 2–13 percent of all transplants, depending on the organ type. While this is a small percentage compared to adults, children have a much longer lifespan ahead of them, resulting in many more years of managing their new organ.

While the morbidities and outcomes of pediatric transplants have been discussed for various organ types, Gupta focused on a general overview of what happens when patients move from pediatric to adult health care. She shared a study examining liver transplant patients who survived about 20 and 25 years after transplantation. The main findings were that survival in children transplanted between ages 11–15 and 15–17 was worse than that of children who were transplanted before their 5th birthday (Ekong et al., 2019). Additionally, older age at transplant was associated with worse patient and graft survival. Gupta also highlighted a study from her center that found increased mortality in children who transferred from pediatric to adult care: one in four young adult liver transplant recipients died after that transition, and she noted that African Americans constituted the majority of these (Katz et al., 2021).

Factors Affecting Outcomes in Pediatric Transplant Recipients

Gupta asked what patient factors should be considered that may adversely affect these outcomes in pediatric transplant recipients. She highlighted the teenage brain, noting it is still very much under construction, with dissociated decision making and strong emotion, even in healthy children. The cerebral abilities that mature latest include foresight, planning, and risk/reward evaluation. Patients with chronic diseases may also have delayed maturation in psychosocial spheres and autonomy. She described the typical adolescent transplant patient: long-term survival is limited, substance abuse peaks, and the suicide rate is tripled. Gupta said that overall, the mortality rate of 18–24-year-olds is twice that of those 12–17, and up to one-third of adolescent transplant patients are nonadherent to medication regimens (Paraskeva et al., 2018). Several studies show risk factors for and causes of nonadherence, including the number of years after transplantation, sex, and parental stress and anxiety, but she noted a risk factor that has been apparent in several studies is a single-parent home, emphasizing the importance of social support (Berquist et al., 2006). Fredericks et al. (2007) showed that functional outcomes include evidence of poor cognitive, intellectual, and health-related QOL after transplantation.

Gupta was optimistic that knowledge of the developing adolescent brain can help providers and caregivers be empathetic and understanding regarding the needs of teenagers and young adults, and thus may facilitate implementation of interventions that support improved functioning in these patients. She highlighted transition programs that support adolescents as they transfer to the adult care setting and place emphasis on individual needs, customized care and treatment, and tracking outcomes. For example,

Gupta shared that her team developed the Adolescent Program 101,[4] which takes a multidisciplinary approach involving providers, patient navigators, social workers, peer support, telemedicine, and other initiatives—and provides intensive monitoring and education as patients transfer to the adult setting.

DISCUSSION

Dorry Segev, associate vice chair of the Department of Surgery at JHU, moderated Session 2. He began by asking the panelists what might contribute to the differences between adult and pediatric survival rates among the various end-organ groups and why some organs show much better pediatric survival when others may even be worse than adult rates. Diaz-Gonzalez de Ferris responded in the context of kidney transplant patients, saying that 10-year posttransplant survival is actually greater for children than adults, but the reason is not completely clear. Some theories include the fewer comorbidities in adolescents and young adults, such as heart disease, diabetes, or lung disease. She also highlighted a study looking at approximately 168,000 transplants across the country up to 55 years old and found that the 14–16-year-old age group—especially those with public insurance and minority status—are at the highest risk of losing their transplanted organ (Andreoni et al., 2013). Gupta agreed, noting similar findings have been seen in liver recipients. She described a study of 25-year outcomes, in which 14–17-year-olds were also the highest risk group (Ekong et al., 2019). Gupta again called attention to the developing adolescent brain and the need for more empathy and support.

Lung transplantation may be unique, said Conrad, because the organ is constantly exposed to the environment, whereas the other organs are generally protected. One concern is that teens join their peer groups and want to do the things they are doing, which can include inhaling substances—even passively. This has especially been more of an issue with the increasing rate of marijuana legalization around the country, Conrad said. Aside from CF patients, she said typically the worse survival rates are not related to recurrence of baseline disease, but she also acknowledged they still do not understand why lungs fibrose. For heart transplants, Chin said adolescent half-lives were quite similar to adults, around 14–15 years, compared to

---

[4] See http://prd-choa.choa.org/medical-services/transplants/adolescent-and-young-adult-program (accessed May 24, 2021).

babies, who have much higher half-lives (25 years). He attributed this to babies being immunologically naïve, compared to older children or adults who are immunologically mature. But he also pointed out that if patients are transplanted as babies, they grew up with posttransplant life as their normal life and are accustomed to all the things that go with it. Chin compared this to a cardiomyopathy patient who may have led a normal life until 16 or 17 and then suddenly becomes sick with numerous new restrictions and obligations; such a patient is more likely to resist recommended treatment regimens, Chin said.

Nonadherence in Children and Adolescents

Segev recalled a study that found that those who had a functioning allograft at age 17 had a 42 percent chance of losing it by the time they were 24 years old (Van Arendonk et al., 2013). During this high-risk window, nearly half of kidney allografts are lost, he said. He asked how the effect of nonadherence with transplant follow-up procedures can be quantified. Segev also asked whether it was possible to quantify the effect on survival rates if nonadherence could be reduced or eliminated. Diaz-Gonzalez de Ferris noted the lack of strong agreement on the definition of nonadherence, so it is difficult to quantify. Another challenge is that patients want to live a normal life, but living with chronic disease is difficult and can be a vicious cycle. For example, in CKD, 30–40 percent of adolescents have attention deficit hyperactivity disorder. They do not perform well in school, do not have great job outlooks, and can have anxiety and depression, as well as high-risk behaviors, which can lead to a vicious cycle that results in nonadherence. They also have employment issues, with nearly half living with their parents, so the experience of growing up and transitioning to adulthood is not the same compared to typical adolescents. Gupta again emphasized the point about single-parent homes contributing to nonadherence, but as children become older, the need for oversight lessens. Additionally, she pointed out a need to reflect racial disparities, and also immune systems differences, when considering nonadherence. Chin added that it is very difficult to quantitate, but there are some possible approaches for detecting nonadherence. For example, drug screenings may be able to help determine whether a patient is following recommended medication regimens.

ASSESSING PHYSICAL, COGNITIVE, AND PSYCHOSOCIAL FUNCTION AFTER ORGAN TRANSPLANTATION IN CHILDREN

As many speakers noted, children face unique challenges as they adjust to their lives following transplantation. In Session 5B regarding physical, cognitive, and psychosocial functioning following transplantation in children, speakers described methods of assessing patient functioning and presented research findings on short- and long-term effects of transplantation on functioning and QOL. A panel discussion further explored the topic of impairments following an organ transplant that can lead to disability in children.

Physical and Cognitive Functioning

Compared to adults, children are transplanted early in life and may have other congenital diseases that cause impairment, but they tend to be quite resilient, said Saeed Mohammad, medical director of pediatric hepatology and liver transplantation at the Northwestern University Feinberg School of Medicine. A critical time of development is affected by transplantation and use of immunosuppressive medications from childhood for many years can also affect the developing brain. Defining functioning can include physical and cognitive realms, where age and pretransplant health status are also important determinants. Functional assessment measures that are age appropriate may be more difficult for children who are chronically ill, because they usually have not attained the milestones expected for certain ages. Ratings may be done by self or proxy (such as a parent), but proxy raters often report more impaired functioning than standardized tests, which tend to underestimate the abilities of children with chronic illnesses, Mohammad explained.

Physical functioning is typically measured through observation of physical ability, such as attaining milestones, the 6-minute walk test, or the Lansky performance scale. Cognitive functioning tools depend on a child's development but could include IQ tests or specific tests of executive functioning and visuospatial abilities. Survey instruments, such as PedsQL or the Patient-Reported Outcomes Measurement Information System scale, could be used for either physical or cognitive functioning. Mohammad presented data on kidney recipients transplanted before the age of 5. Poor developmental outcomes were associated with long-term dialysis, and with hemodialysis (Popel et al., 2019). Kidney transplant recipients had lower visual-motor integration, full-scale IQ, and general adaptive composite scores. A separate study of heart transplant patients compared those with CHD to those who had a failing heart. Despite all of them having been transplant recipients at a very young age, the patients with CHD scored lower (Urschel et al., 2018). He highlighted the differences between the two groups, noting that those with CHD have more surgeries, greater kidney injury, and more days in the ICU, demonstrating the significance of the course of illness before transplantation in addition to other factors.

Liver recipients also had cognitive functioning studied. Mohammad shared one study of a multicenter trial across three time points that showed both cognitive functioning and school functioning decreased over time. The study suggested that more than half of the adolescents with liver transplants may be at risk of poor school functioning (Ohnemus et al., 2020). Mohammad said this could also be because as patients transition into high school, they may have difficulty adjusting to the increased demands on their brains' executive functioning.

When discussing areas for improvement, Mohammad noted that physical functioning in children is closest to normal in liver and kidney recipients, but heart recipients are the most at risk for functional deficits. Pediatric heart patients are generally transplanted at a young age and are very ill before transplantation. They also typically have lower oxygen levels, which may affect their cognitive outcomes. Cognitive functioning may also worsen with age due to the increased need for executive functioning. Regarding knowledge gaps and possible interventions for improving functional outcomes, he identified a need for functional assessment measures collected in real time to enhance the identification of modifiable factors. Mohammad explained that existing measures identify a problem but cannot indicate when it occurred (before transplantation or around the time of surgery), making it difficult to know how best to intervene to improve outcomes. Real-time assessment measures might help overcome this barrier, he said.

Psychosocial Risk Factors Associated with Transplant Outcomes in Children

Eyal Shemesh, chief of the Division of Developmental and Behavioral Pediatrics at Mount Sinai Kravis Children's Hospital, emphasized that children are not just small adults. They have different trajectories and somewhat different risks following transplantation. Pediatric transplantation is best viewed as a lifesaving transition from a deadly risk to a chronic illness, he said, echoing previous comments, but it is not a cure that brings children to full health. Transplantation means a lifelong commitment to immunosuppression management. While the outcome is often a long and productive life, Shemesh said transplantation can lead to many complications and this is especially true with children who may live with a transplant the majority of their lives.

Emphasizing that that cognitive impairment is an important concern in children, Shemesh said that a large percentage of pediatric transplant patients have schooling difficulties. Based on his research—mainly on a liver transplant prospective child cohort assessed 1 year after transplant—Shemesh indicated that psychosocial demographic challenges were top predictors of risk. He shared the following predictors of cognitive impairment, cautioning that they are not necessarily causal but only indicate a risk:

- History of child abuse
- Single-parent household
- Zip code (often a proxy for low socioeconomic status)
- Race (African American)
- Sex (female, especially predictive in adolescent populations)

Monitoring is very important, continued Shemesh, including adherence to medical recommendations, which is something that is unique to transplant patients. Transplant patients must take immunosuppressive medications consistently for the rest of their lives. Monitoring school functioning is also important, given the cognitive impairment risks. Shemesh shared data from a liver transplant child cohort study showing that in adolescents, 53 percent who were nonadherent had a rejection episode, compared to just 6 percent of those who were adherent (Shemesh et al., 2017). He said awareness of the risk of nonadherence is a step toward mitigating it. Because children can change as they grow and develop, assessments and evaluations need to be repeated again and again, especially during adolescence, so the level of risk can be proactively addressed. Shemesh stressed that in the young transplant population, all family members need support, not just the patient. He added that resources for additional support should be allocated for patients who are at high risk, with special attention to the prevalence of PTSD and depression.

DISCUSSION

Lease and Rogal co-moderated the discussion. Lease first asked Mohammad how effective cognitive interventions are at improving cognitive function in children and how it might vary based on the underlying causes of the decline. He replied that in general, most kids are transplanted quite early, before they turn 5, so there is not a lot of testing before transplantation. It can also be difficult to differentiate complications that happen after transplantation from something that was part of the underlying disease. He referred to the example of recipients with CHD having worse cognitive outcomes compared to those with other types of heart disease, and he said they see the same thing in liver recipients. Patients with metabolic diseases that can affect the whole body struggle more than those with other liver ailments.

Turning to Shemesh, Lease wondered how long after transplantation would anyone be able to generally see the apex of functioning in children. Shemesh responded he did not think of functioning as a linear trajectory. He envisions function as a "seesaw" or something that is coming and going, which is why it is most important to monitor progress or decline. In addition to the risk period of adolescence, he said, studies of long-term trajectory show a risk period in adulthood.

Regarding what might be specifically beneficial for children, Mohammad cited a need for resources to monitor their physical, cognitive, and psychosocial development, but said such resources are not always easily available. For example, clinicians may refer a child who is struggling to a therapist or psychologist, but it is often up to the family to find someone, which can be very difficult. That provider also may not be well versed in the specific challenges transplant recipients face, which might include PTSD from hospitalization, difficulty adhering to medication regimens, or the vulnerability that may come from being different from other children. This is definitely an area that could benefit from more easily accessible resources, he stated. Shemesh added that children are naturally completely dependent on their parents, but in cases where the parent is not completely functional, then it may necessary to create an environment around the child that can help them thrive, regardless of their situation.

In terms of monitoring those who are not able to access regular health care, Shemesh said the COVID-19 era catapulted them into remote monitoring more quickly than he could have imagined. He is working on research to show the efficacy of these remote appointments, which would inherently remove the burden of traveling to the clinic. He also described multiple apps that try to interact with patients to have them check in with their care team and communicate directly with the care team if something is going wrong or they have questions.

One thing about adult transplantation programs, said Lease, is that they do not have the same structure or resources built into them as the pediatric programs do. She asked for suggestions for adult transplantation programs that are now taking care of pediatric patients who have transitioned into their care. Shemesh said it may help if programs focus on not only the adult side but also the pediatric side. As young patients approach a transition to adult care, he suggested a separate transition program may ensure pediatric patients are ready for the next stage of care by helping them to build self-sufficiency. Mohammad added that the volume of pediatric patients is smaller compared to adults, so it is difficult for adult programs to mimic everything that is done. Lease noted that adolescence is very vulnerable, and she cautioned against losing the opportunity for them to maintain their progress.

Rogal commented on the fine line between monitoring adherence and blaming the patients, as adherence is not merely related to motivation and may be influenced by systemic barriers. Shemesh agreed, saying he had studied adherence in both adults and children, but children may have a better chance to benefit from adherence interventions because they often have a parent or other partner that can be involved. He advocated for specifically targeting resources instead of trying to make sure that everyone in the clinic gets everything available, because some patients will have much more of a need. The resources could include social workers, psychologists, or physicians, but it depends on the case. Shemesh noted that the largest predictor of nonadherence in their cohort was child abuse, a horrific intersection with transplantation (Shemesh et al., 2007). Mohammad added that tailoring the services to the population is necessary, agreeing that some patients need more help and reminders to adhere to the treatment schedules. He also highlighted the importance of understanding family situations, using the example of housing instability. If medications need to be refrigerated but patients cannot consistently comply, they are not able to take the medications as prescribed. Understanding each family's position as to why this happens is important, he said, and so is the need to be sensitive to the stigma associated with things such as being unable to afford medications.

Lease asked if there were special SSA considerations when the child is receiving disability benefits and is in the child welfare system. Shemesh acknowledged he did not know SSA considerations specifically but argued that those children who are in the transplant system need more resources to support their health and QOL. Mohammad agreed they are a higher-risk population and could be monitored more closely and provided with more resources earlier after transplantation.

A final question was about posttransplant functioning after adolescence, based on the level of adherence during adolescence, for those patients who survive into young adulthood. Shemesh noted the selection bias, because the only outcomes to examine would be in patients who did survive that tumultuous period. In addition, he said there is some indication in the literature that if patients make it through the vulnerable period of adolescence, they can improve afterward. But, Shemesh added, many patients do not make it through a period of adolescent nonadherence. Mohammad said for survivors, there may be no long-term effects on functioning, though they may lose a grade in school depending on how long they are hospitalized. But others may end up with diminished graft function, so the effects on functioning would be related to the number of medications and which side effects might be playing a role. Mohammad said that overall outcomes for pediatric patients are very good for liver, kidney, and heart transplants. They likely need close monitoring, and some will require more support, but he believed it is something that can be overcome for them to live a fairly normal life. Shemesh agreed, adding that the focus on the family unit when considering needs and outcomes for children is incredibly important, as any child will not do well when a parent is not well.

5

Treatments, Technologies, and Interventions Affecting Function After Transplantation

Transplantation is a complex procedure that requires sophisticated technology, advanced surgical and medical expertise, and specialized care management. Session 4 of the workshop focused on the medical and supportive interventions patients may need to mitigate or treat possible organ rejection or failure, infections, illness, and impaired function. Speakers described the pharmacologic treatments and their side effects following transplantation and described the standard and emerging practices to support and improve health and functioning, including prehabilitation, posttransplant rehabilitation, and palliative care. The last section highlights the panel discussion, including salient questions asked by attendees from SSA, and suggestions from individual speakers for taking these approaches to the next level.

PRETRANSPLANT CARE MANAGEMENT

Mara McAdams-DeMarco, director of clinical and outcomes research at JHU, described the negative outcomes impacted by pretransplant impairments. For example, mortality and graft loss risk are elevated when patients have pretransplant conditions, such as frailty, walking or cognitive impairments, obesity, or unintentional weight loss. She explained that among kidney recipients, those who had a walking impairment prior to transplantation were found to have a mortality rate three times higher than those who did not (Thomas et al., 2020). For this population, intervening prior to transplantation—often referred to as prehabilitation—is a way of increasing the probability of successful transplantation. Surgery is a significant physiologic stressor, causing changes in the body, such as stress hormone production and increased inflammation, and can be comparable to intense exercise. McAdams-DeMarco said prehabilitation interventions are designed to enhance the functional capacity to tolerate the stress of surgery and will typically include exercise components and sometimes nutritional or psychological components. This approach allows the care team to shift the focus to optimization prior to surgery instead of rehabilitation afterward, she said. Transplantation represents an ideal setting for this approach, she added, because people often wait long periods for a transplant and during this time suffer from aging, frailty, or other comorbidities. McAdams-DeMarco presented a conceptual model of prehabilitation where multiple components are brought together with a goal of improving long-term outcomes (see Figure 5-1).

McAdams-DeMarco explained that candidates may be more motivated to start a new program before transplantation. Because patients often experience a variety of other challenges following the procedure, they may find it easier to modify their daily routine prior to the transplant. She added that many patients have prolonged recovery and may be rehospitalized in

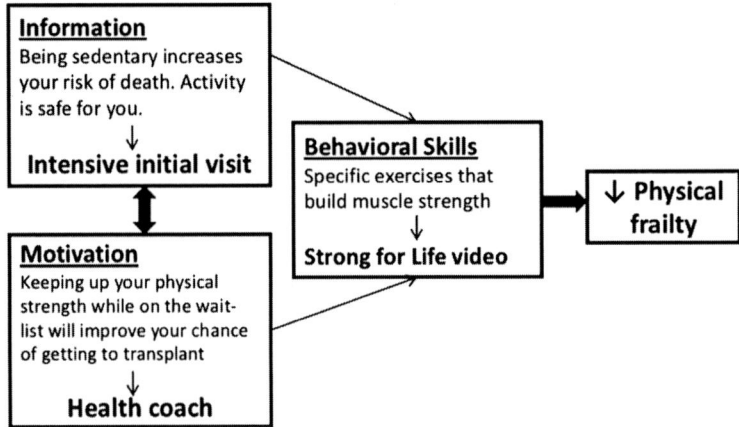

FIGURE 5-1 Three components of the strength training interventions for liver transplant patients based on the Information-Motivation-Behavioral Skills conception model for modifying individual health behaviors.
SOURCES: Mara McAdams-DeMarco presentation, March 23, 2021; Lai et al., 2021.

the early postoperative period, so this is difficult time to try new things—especially activities that add stress to the body.

A prehabilitation program such as this can have several different types of interventions or approaches. McAdams-DeMarco shared several examples across different organ types. For lung transplant candidates, pulmonary prehabilitation is the most common. She summarized different studies looking at this intervention and noted that while duration and exercise type differed by study, all studies reported improved exercise capacity and QOL following the interventions (Florian et al., 2013; Li et al., 2013). Other studies of lung transplant candidates looked at home-based prehabilitation using mobile technology, which also allows patients to track their progress. Others have examined home-based exercise and saw improvements in 6-minute walk distance for more than one-quarter of participants. This intervention was associated with improved posttransplant outcomes, including less time on mechanical ventilation and reduced length of hospital and ICU stay (Massierer et al., 2020). McAdams-DeMarco reported that some studies in liver transplant candidates found smartphone apps to be effective in increasing physical performance, while other studies have demonstrated home-based programs focusing on exercise and strength training were safe and improved QOL. She described her own study of prehabilitation for kidney transplants: 40-minute therapy sessions with a goal of tailoring the program to improve physical functioning by performing cardiovascular exercises (McAdams-DeMarco et al., 2019). Patients noted in feedback that 100 percent were very satisfied with the prehabilitation and overall were very positive, saying that it helped them to sustain endurance, maintain better weight control, and even improve their attitude coming into transplantation. She shared data showing a 64 percent improvement in physical activity over 2 months. Only five candidates went on to receive their transplant during the study, but McAdams-DeMarco noted that their hospital length of stay was reduced by 5 days (McAdams-DeMarco et al., 2019).

In conclusion, McAdams-DeMarco highlighted the knowledge gaps regarding pretransplant interventions. She said that while the pretransplant period is an ideal window to recruit patients into efforts to modify their behavior that will benefit overall health following transplantation, the challenge is that there are only two studies of transplant candidates (lung and kidney, respectively) showing that prehabilitation can affect posttransplant outcomes. She described a need for future research to identify the optimal transplant patient population, define a standard prehabilitation program, identify optimal timing and duration of interventions, and quantify costs.

Answering these questions will help to answer whether prehabilitation improves pre- and posttransplant outcomes and prevents impairments that can lead to disability, McAdams-DeMarco said.

PHARMACOLOGIC TREATMENTS AFTER TRANSPLANTATION

Solid organ transplantation is major surgery with a variable length of recovery and duration of inpatient stay, said Saeed Mohammad, medical director of pediatric hepatology and liver transplantation at the Northwestern University Feinberg School of Medicine. At discharge, transplant patients may be taking more than 10 medications; their number and nature can make recovery more or less difficult and affect physical, emotional, cognitive, and social functioning. In assessments of functioning, it is important to compare functioning to previous ability as well as healthy controls. Mohammad cited various methods of measurement, including questionnaires, active methods, such as treadmills, or observer measures, such as interviews by trained personnel or parental observation. Finally, imaging methods exist, such as functional MRI to measure how the brain uses energy when participating in a certain task and computed tomography scans to measure muscle mass.

In the short term, or the first 3 months after transplantation, a number of different medications may affect functioning, he said. Narcotics used for pain relief can lead to decreased physical and cognitive functioning. Patients are also often on antibiotics or antiviral medications, which can cause nausea and diarrhea. Transplant recipients need to take immunosuppressive medications for life to prevent organ rejection, but these medications can often cause neurological symptoms that may affect physical and cognitive functioning. Tacrolimus is the most commonly used immunosuppressive medication, Mohammad explained. Tacrolimus can cause tremors, dizziness, anemia, or insomnia. Longer-term effects may include diabetes and cardiovascular disease, which can both affect neurological functioning.

Mohammad presented a study looking at changes in body composition after liver transplant comparing two different medications. Patients on cyclosporine had an increase in lean muscle mass and more significant decrease in fat index compared to patients on tacrolimus, showing that different medications can affect body composition in unique ways, which can lead to long-term effects (Brito-Costa et al., 2016). Pflugrad et al. (2020) examine cognitive functioning, comparing kidney recipients assessed at 1,

5, and 10 years after transplantation to liver recipients and healthy controls. All transplant recipients scored lower than healthy controls across the measured domains: immediate memory, visuospatial/constructional, language, attention, and delayed memory (see Figure 5-2). He noted that language and delayed memory domains remained the most normal.

Corticosteroids are another class of medications used in transplants for a long time. They can cause weight gain, mood disturbances, and bone demineralization, which can affect long-term physical functioning. Mycophenolate is a widely used antimetabolite medication to prevent organ rejection. However, Mohammad explained that it can cause abdominal pain, nausea, diarrhea, and anemia. He presented a study where patients were taking mycophenolate, but one group of patients were given a different form (an enteric-coated formulation) that resulted in less nausea and less abdominal pain. While it was a small study, he showed that many of the functioning measures all improved in 8 weeks just by changing the route of administration, demonstrating how small changes in treatment

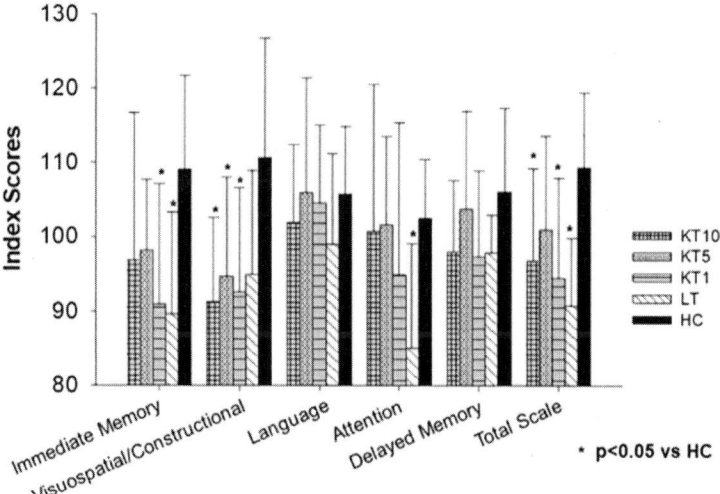

FIGURE 5-2 Brain function and metabolism in patients with long-term tacrolimus therapy after kidney transplantation compared to patients after liver transplantation and healthy controls.
NOTE: HC = healthy control; KT1 = 1 year post-kidney transplantation; KT5 = 5 years post-kidney transplantation; KT10 = 10 years post-kidney transplantation; LT = liver transplantation.
SOURCES: Saeed Mohammad presentation, March 23, 2021; Pflugrad et al., 2020.

regimen can greatly improve functioning (Langone et al., 2011). Finally, because hypertension can affect many patients after transplantation, antihypertensive drugs have been known to cause dizziness, headache, constipation, and fatigue.

Mohammad commented on the indirect side effects of these medications. First is the perception of vulnerability, as many patients may feel quite vulnerable following the transplant and may be more likely to limit their physical activity because they are worried about getting hurt. Patients can also feel very dependent on medications and experience stress and anxiety in trying to maintain medication levels and adhere to the right schedule. For children, he said, the physical side effects of weight gain or hair loss can also be difficult to cope with and may lead to bullying, which affects their emotional and social functioning. In conclusion, Mohammad suggested that medications used in transplantation can have unwanted side effects, and these have to be routinely monitored and managed to optimize short- and long-term functioning after transplant surgery.

REHABILITATION AFTER TRANSPLANTATION

Sunita Mathur, associate professor and physical therapist at the University of Toronto, presented on posttransplant rehabilitation. The primary goal of this intervention is not only to increase survival of those with severe organ disease, she said, but also to improve patients' QOL. Many transplant recipients do not enjoy the full benefits of organ transplantation and are not able to reach their expected level of physical function—which then affects their ability to resume personal or societal roles, such as functioning as a family caregiver or employee. The goals of posttransplant rehabilitation are multifaceted and thus require a multidisciplinary approach. Beyond physical functioning, rehabilitation goals can also include improving treatment adherence, addressing sleep quality, addressing mental health issues, and providing social support, such as a peer network for the recipient and their family. Across all organ groups, Mathur noted that aerobic exercise capacity and muscle strength are reduced for the majority of patients. This is likely caused by the extended periods of bedrest and immobility before and after transplantation. Additionally, early medical complications after transplantation may require hospitalization, which can impact the ability to return to typical daily activities. Given the number of immunosuppressive medications required, as described by Mohammad, numerous long-term effects may cause complications and affect physical functioning.

To address the spectrum of needs that most transplant patients have, which include the need for support with physical functioning, treatment adherence, sleep quality, mental health, and social support, Mathur said the rehabilitation process should occur throughout the continuum of care—from the acute care hospital setting to the early phases after transplantation. Mathur explained that early-phase rehabilitation is the most well described in the literature, especially in terms of exercise training, but there is no set structure for posttransplant rehabilitation overall. Mathur described the rehabilitation approach at the Toronto Lung Transplant Program, where recipients have prehabilitation (as discussed by McAdams-DeMarco) for the duration of their waiting period, and then immediately following the operation, they are actively seen by physical therapists in the ICU for early mobility and exercise to increase functioning and independence. After discharge, there is a mandatory outpatient exercise program for 3 months after transplantation. Patients who are not ready for outpatient programs can be discharged to an inpatient program to address medical needs or functional limitations. After this 3-month period, she described the regular follow-up of patients and ongoing counseling from physical therapists that occurs.

Examining outcomes for these types of programs, Mathur said that most knowledge comes from studies on exercise training. Her team recently published a systematic review and meta-analysis on the effects of exercise training across solid-organ transplant groups. They found great improvements across all organ types seen in aerobic exercise capacity, such as leg muscle strength and QOL, all resulting from regular exercise training (Janaudis-Ferreira et al., 2021). They also found some evidence of improved cardiovascular health and emerging evidence for improvements in mental health outcomes, such as depression and anxiety, but she stressed that more research is needed.

More than just clinical outcomes are important to consider, said Mathur. She shared a study of lung recipients that found those in the exercise program perceived it to be a highly valuable tool to assist them in returning to normal life while providing the motivation and peer support needed to achieve their own desired level of physical performance (Fuller et al., 2014). Mathur highlighted a study her team conducted in which they surveyed solid organ recipients and found that all who attended the rehabilitation program found it beneficial to their health and well-being (Schoo et al., 2017). Several factors were at play, but patients who had poorer health or were experiencing symptoms were less likely to attend the program. While evidence is now established for the needs and benefits of these rehabilitation programs, she noted the limitations in availability of programs that patients can access.

Mathur called attention to the gaps in current knowledge and potential future directions for research. A multidisciplinary approach to rehabilitation is needed to address the full spectrum of needs beyond exercise training, she said. Greater availability of programs specific to different transplant recipients and greater inquiry into the methods of delivery for these programs are also needed. It can be difficult for hospital-based programs to be the only option for rehabilitation for recipients, particularly in the long term. Given the increase in available technology and virtual systems, patients can also participate from home, which would reduce many barriers for attending in-person programs. Further evidence for long-term outcomes of rehabilitation, including QOL and survival outcomes, need to be determined to understand morbidity and mortality rates. Finally, Mathur called for reducing barriers for physician counseling around exercise and rehabilitation because their endorsement is such an important factor influencing patients' behavior. She suggested disseminating evidence-based guidelines and the evidence of benefits to both physicians and patients of various rehabilitation programs.

PALLIATIVE CARE

To give a better understanding of palliative care, Kirsten Wentlandt of the Ajmera Transplant Centre at the University Health Network in Toronto provided a definition from the World Health Organization (see Box 5-1). It describes a philosophy of care that is focused on QOL, to support patients facing a life-threatening illness and assist their caregivers and families. While patients may not necessarily be acutely dying, palliative care focuses on preventing and relieving suffering and managing physical, psychological, and spiritual aspects of care. Palliative care does not intend to hasten or postpone death, Wentlandt explained, and most palliative care studies show no change at all in mortality rates compared to typical medical care. But, she added, a few studies have shown that patients can live longer when integrating palliative care (Temel et al., 2010). Palliative care is applicable early in the disease course and does not have to be mutually exclusive with life-prolonging care. Instead, Wentlandt said that in 99 percent of her work, she focuses on supporting patients alongside other care providers while they are awaiting transplantation or still undergoing therapies to prolong life.

> **BOX 5-1**
> **Definition of Palliative Care**
>
> "An approach that improves QOL of patients and their families facing the problems associated with life-threatening illness, through the prevention and relief of suffering by means of early identification and impeccable assessment and treatment of pain and other problems, physical, psychological and spiritual."
>
> SOURCES: Kirsten Wentlandt presentation, March 23, 2021; WHO, 2020.

In her overview of the field, Wentlandt presented a model of four main aspects of palliative care and common outcomes that follow palliative care integration (see Box 5-2). In addition to optimizing symptom management, she said palliative care specialists help the patient and family with advance care planning and decisions about the health care they want to receive. Care coordination is also important, she said, as various providers across the continuum, from transplant specialists at tertiary level hospitals to community-

> **BOX 5-2**
> **Elements of Palliative Care and Common Outcomes**
>
> 1. Optimal symptom management: decreased symptom burden, decreased depression and anxiety, improved patient satisfaction, and improved QOL
> 2. Support of family: decreased caregiver burden, decreased depression and anxiety, and improved caregiver satisfaction
> 3. Advance care planning: improved frequency of conversations about care goals and increased the likelihood of providing goal concordant care
> 4. Care coordination: decreased emergency room visits, decreased hospital admissions, improved lengths of stay, decreased ICU care, and decreased health care costs
>
> SOURCES: Kirsten Wentlandt presentation, March 23, 2021; Bajwah et al., 2020; Gonzalez-Jaramillo et al., 2020; Quinn et al., 2020.

based providers, are working as a team to support patients' goals of care and to ensure their alignment with the provision of clinical care.

Looking at the research on the subject, including two recently published systematic reviews, Wentlandt said that overall, the findings demonstrate that palliative care provides an improvement in symptom burden—both physical and mental health symptoms—and in patient satisfaction and QOL (Bajwah et al., 2020; Gonzalez-Jaramillo et al., 2020). Studies have also found decreased caregiver burden, improved depression and anxiety scores, and improved caregiver satisfaction. Other benefits were decreased emergency room visits and hospital admissions, decreased length of hospital stays and ICU care, and reduced health care and end-of-life hospitalization costs. Much of this work stems from research in cancer populations, she explained, but the past decade has seen an integration of palliative care into other populations (Quinn et al., 2020). Evidence is now emerging of very similar benefits for different types of patients, such as transplant recipients.

Despite the research showing that patients with advanced organ disease, like organ recipients, can have symptom burdens as high as or higher than patients with cancer, rates of integration of palliative care for patients with organ failure are quite low around the world (Pantilat et al., 2012). Wentlandt noted that only about 10–30 percent of palliative care referrals made for hospitalized patients in the United States are for those with organ failure (Schoenherr et al., 2019). In addition, she said patients with organ failure are largely underrepresented in data on hospice deaths. Additionally, when patients with organ failure are referred to palliative care or hospice, it is often days or even hours before death. Digging deeper into available research, she explained that only about 20 studies looked at palliative care integration in transplant populations. But even with this small number, recurrent themes of positive benefits exist, including reduced symptom burden, decreased anxiety and depression, and improvement in patient satisfaction and QOL (Gustafson and Song, 2020). They have also shown improvement in goal-concordant care, or understanding what patients want and documenting it in their charts. Importantly, she argued that early evidence supports palliative care specialists working with patients at all stages in their transplant journey.

As an example of the need for palliative care with this specific patient population, Wentlandt highlighted a large recent study in the United States that looked at more than 500,000 patients who died from ESRD (Butler et al., 2020). It specifically examined patients who were exposed to transplant, whether listed and waitlisted or assessed and not listed, including those who went on to get a transplant and those who died while waiting. Simply being exposed to transplant, compared to patients who were not, resulted in a significant increase in ICU admissions, aggressive interventions at end of life, increased likelihood of dying in a hospital, and lower likelihood of being connected to palliative care and hospice. She said these patients may have benefited from a targeted conversation to understand whether this type of care was what they really wanted. She argued for a more thoughtful approach to palliative care integration in transplant populations, especially knowing now that these patients are very unlikely to receive this care without transplant programs taking proactive steps to remedy this.

DISCUSSION

Dorry Segev and Hannah Valantine moderated a discussion on medical and supportive interventions following organ transplantation. They began by asking how widely prehabilitation is currently used in the transplant community and whether it is considered a best practice. McAdams-DeMarco said that it might be studied as part of a research protocol, but she was not aware of any transplant centers that prescribe it as part of their program. However, she added that many centers have expressed interest in providing prehabilitation but have many questions about who is involved and when, where, and how it takes place, as well as how much it costs and who pays for it, which are still unanswered.

In response to a question on the relation of QOL measures after transplantation to survival rates, Mathur explained that QOL sometimes has a different trajectory than survival. However, she did report progressive or acute changes in functional ability leading to organ rejection and mortality. One simple measure that can be predictive of overall wellness is strength of lower extremity muscles, particularly quadriceps strength. She said these simple functional measures can be very good predictors for mortality or rejection but are not the only thing contributing to QOL, as it is influenced by many different factors. Adding the pediatric perspective, Mohammad said QOL generally improves after transplantation, but it does hit a plateau in teenage years and often falls short of the normal population's average QOL. Why this is the case is not understand, he explained, as labs are normal and biochemically the organs are working, but they just do not hit that optimal QOL measure. Bringing in research on frailty, McAdams-DeMarco said that frail patients experience significant improvement in posttransplant health-related QOL, cognitive function, and overall functioning. Wentlandt added that a lot of QOL scores or measures are related to patient expectations. QOL measures are very subjective, so even if patients are doing well clinically, they might be taking many more medications, have more hospital visits, or be attached to a device, which can all act as barriers to their QOL and visions for the future. But, she said, sometimes even just a simple conversation acknowledging suffering or the need to adjust goals and focus can have a big effect on QOL. Transplantation is also a palliative intervention, because patients are exchanging one illness for another chronic illness, hoping to improve survival but ultimately QOL.

Valantine also asked what proportion of recipients has access to late-phase rehabilitation and how long that access usually lasts. Mathur used her transplant center's experience as an example and said they have a mandatory pretransplant rehabilitation program for all lung transplant candidates. Mathur noted that this is an excellent program but is not indicative of standard practices across all transplant centers. Often, it can be left up to the patient to find a program if they need one—many will find a peer support network or meet up with other patients for walks or cycling.

Finally, Segev asked whether exercise training is a viable rehabilitation option for everyone or just a certain subgroup. McAdams-DeMarco replied that prehabilitation is an important intervention for all transplant patients, and the pretransplant period is a great opportunity to get people up and moving and have them start new healthy routines. It is also a chance to have them do whatever it is they are capable of doing, which can help recuperation and recovery after their very important surgical intervention. Mathur agreed that it would also be an important intervention in the posttransplant rehabilitation phase that would be beneficial to everyone, regardless of initial physical condition. However, several factors can affect a person's ability to improve, one of which is the challenge of immunosuppression and how that can affect muscles. She said transplant recipients have often reported that these medications affect how the muscle regenerates and adapts to exercise, with some feeling like they hit a wall at a certain point and are not capable of making any more improvements. But generally, Mathur said, most people can achieve the goals they desire, and exercise training as a rehabilitation program should be made available to all recipients regardless of their current level of activity.

When asked about predictions for the state of the science on palliative care, such as the ability to work virtually or integrate robotics to assist medical professionals, Wentlandt answered that the COVID-19 pandemic has shown that a lot of palliative care can be done virtually. She said many patients consider virtual meetings a helpful option because it is not always necessary to travel in order to connect. However, she did not see a place for robots or autonomous devices in the important and sometimes emotional conversations with patients that she does regularly. They might be able to help with charting or review of some patient information, but she cautioned that successful interactions with patients are often an exchange of both verbal and nonverbal cues between patients and their providers and this is something that might be missed without a familiar, human interaction.

Valantine asked how to get many of these approaches more widely adopted and whether there is a need for more research, funding, or something else. McAdams-DeMarco acknowledged there is a need to define the ideal prehabilitation program for each of the solid organ transplant candidates that can be customized for individuals. She suggested this could be done through research and quality improvement efforts. Wentlandt noted the dearth of research on palliative care in the transplant field and suggested more prospective long-term studies that follow patients that undergo this type of care during transplant to document any benefits. Better integration of palliative care in transplant centers would also be helpful, Wentlandt said, as it currently can be variable depending on the location or type of organ. To garner more support for exercise-based prehabilitation, and eventually forming guidelines to allow physicians to feel comfortable making recommendations, Mathur suggested more randomized controlled trials. Mathur also said there is not much information about the health care economics of delivering this type of intervention and whether it is cost effective. Finally, there is the question of how prehabilitation affects survival and whether prehabilitation can reduce the risk of comorbidities following transplantation. All of these questions would be very helpful to have more insight on, she said, but do require longitudinal studies. From a pharmacologic perspective, Mohammad was interested in ways to minimize side effects from some of the medications. Additionally, a study of reimbursement of prehabilitation and rehabilitation programs would be beneficial. It can be difficult for patients to find a rehabilitation center due to both the scarcity of available programs and insurance coverage frequently refusing to cover the cost. Both public and private insurance companies typically pay for surgery and reimburse the transplant center well, he said, but the rehabilitation required is often not covered by health plans and patients are unable to pay out of pocket.

6

Future Outlook for Organ Transplantation and Disability

The workshop discussions covered the complexity of organ transplantation and recovery and the added challenges of incorporating this knowledge into the world of SSA disability determinations and ongoing reviews. Sara Rosenbaum of The George Washington University and James Bowman of the Health Resources and Services Administration moderated a final discussion, allowing for reflection and expert perspectives across topics. Panelists included Aditi Gupta, University of Kansas Medical Center; Erika Lease, University of Washington; Jignesh Patel, Cedars-Sinai Medical Center; and Tanjala Purnell, JHU.

Bowman summarized what the speakers covered during the workshop sessions, first noting that there is no typical transplant patient, as each one is unique and has a different and varied experience. This can relate to many QOL expectations and the goals clinicians might have for themselves or their patients. Decades ago, he said, if a clinician kept a patient alive and they had a functioning organ, the clinician had succeeded. But at this point, the field has grown and improved and now gone beyond those expectations, so it is necessary to really listen to what patients want out of life afterward. Related to this, Bowman said, is that the U.S. health "system" is really many systems, requiring high levels of case coordination, which can leave patients vulnerable to gaps in care and services during the handoffs across systems. He added that dedicated case management can improve many of the challenges for transplant recipients.

In addition, Bowman remarked that COVID-19 has shown the vast potential for using technologies such as telehealth and remote appointments, and it compelled providers and systems to adapt to approaches that successfully manage patients from miles away. Lastly, Bowman commented on the issue of disparities in transplantation and spoke of a need to target patients and populations more precisely to better provide solutions, ideally mitigating some of the poor outcomes related to disparities.

COVID-19-RELATED CONCERNS FOR TRANSPLANT PATIENTS

Bowman posed a question of whether evidence exists regarding the interaction of recipients who have recovered from COVID-19 but still have residual effects in organ function—more systematically or for either their transplant organ or long-term recovery. Lease responded that there are two ways of viewing this question—thinking about those who have yet to undergo transplant and those who have received a new organ. In a handful of cases where transplant recipients had COVID-19, while the acute infection resolved, they never fully recovered and then developed acute respiratory distress syndrome.[1] Another cohort is emerging of patients who may recover enough to leave the hospital but have permanent lung damage requiring a future transplant. However, clarity about other systemic effects of COVID-19 is still lacking, she said, and how it might affect the ability to even get to transplantation or do well after transplantation. Researchers are also trying to understand how COVID-19 affects recipients, and some registries are trying to collect this data right now. Researchers still do not know a great deal, said Lease, but a lot of people are looking at these questions and hope to have more answers.

Patel responded that even before transplantation, patients acquiring COVID-19 faced challenges, as they may test positive for several weeks after the initial infection, but it is unknown how safe it is yet for them to proceed with the transplant and immunosuppressive medications regimen, he said. Another problem is that many potential donors now have a history of COVID-19, died from it, or tested positive prior to organ procurement. As Lease mentioned, whether it is safe to receive organs from such donors is still unknown, but it is an area of active investigation. Numerous recipients have also been infected with COVID-19 after transplantation, and

---

[1] At the time of the workshop in March 2021.

the data from the past year show that transplant patients do not do very well. Mortality rates have been as high as 25 percent once a patient is hospitalized, Patel stated. But he highlighted a large registry being built at the University of Washington for all solid organ transplant patients who have contracted COVID-19, so they are continuing to learn from that data. His final issue was that of vaccines; though they have been proven very effective at preventing hospitalization and death in the normal healthy population, evidence is increasing that transplant recipients may not mount the same antibody response, causing anxiety and concern among patients.

Gupta mentioned the complexity of managing acute COVID-19 in the transplant population given their intentional immunosuppression. COVID-19, she said, can induce an inflammatory cascade, and the immunosuppressive medications could actually slow the cascade. But additional questions remain surrounding how to direct or continue treatments during an active infection. Commenting on vaccines, she discussed the plasmapheresis that can occur as part of the treatment for rejection. Vaccinated patients who receive plasmapheresis will probably have their antibodies removed, she said, but experts are not sure if these patients should receive another dose of vaccine.

Rosenbaum, shifting to the topic of outcomes, posed a question with two dimensions in mind—technique and equity. She asked what the biggest impediments are to improving survival times and functional ability for transplant recipients. Specifically, she said, this should not only include the technical breakthroughs, but, given the discussion around disparities, should also consider the access to such breakthroughs and what that may look like for different populations. Purnell responded that the 5- to 10-year mark after transplant is when they start to see greater gaps in disparities. She noted that historically, this is also around the time when people have lost their Medicare coverage for immunosuppressive medications. Purnell expressed excitement about new legislation being considered that would improve longer-term coverage for those drugs but mentioned the reason to think about other basic human needs. For example, COVID-19 has inspired a lot of emphasis on keeping a safe distance from others who may present more of a risk for the virus, but she asked what that means for patients who do not have homes where they can safely isolate. Additionally, Purnell stated that returning to work may illuminate important questions about protections in place for transplant recipients who want to contribute to society. This needs to go beyond written policies, she said, to also include operational guidance for employees, such as whom they should call if they feel they are not able to safely perform their job duties. Not everyone can work remotely, so what are the consequences in the case of patients who may be lower-wage essential workers, she asked.

EMERGING TECHNOLOGIES TO WATCH

Rosenbaum asked what emerging technologies people are following closely and what kind of timeline people should expect for new and promising features in the field to become standard practice. Patel highlighted the challenges of conducting clinical trials because the number of patients with certain conditions is small and each program has a limited set of patients. Despite advances in certain areas that have been shown to be effective, getting patients covered by insurance has been a big challenge. Therapies from other areas, such as autoimmune diseases, are potentially useful, but researchers are still looking at this transition to see how it might best work. Patel called attention to the need for better monitoring for rejection without being invasive, such as through blood tests, which is an area of active investigation. Finally, he noted the evolution that the field is continuing to undergo, especially in terms of genetically engineering animals to provide a source of organs for humans. While this has been an area of research for decades, it may become reality in the next few years. Gupta noted the time differences in innovations; research on drugs and artificial organs may take longer, but other practical changes and developments could be moved along more quickly—such as exercise and nutrition programs. She also pointed to medications and more systemic barriers, saying if financial and other access barriers can be broken, some patients could see immediate benefit.

Lease described the field of lung transplantation as much smaller and with less volume of transplants. The field has tried to borrow from other organ research, such as kidney studies. Not all organ transplant recipients are the same, and interventions across organ types are not easily generalizable, so some interventions that may work for one type may not work for another. She agreed with the importance of innovations that are less invasive and that can be done from afar, without requiring travel to the transplant center. Lease also noted that because lung transplant patients require so much immunosuppression compared to other organ recipients, they are limited by the complications due to these medications. Purnell also highlighted the advances in reimbursement for virtual visits over the past year. She explained that they have been able to close some gaps in care coordination and figure out very quickly how to get experts to speak at grand rounds nationwide to be sources of information virtually. From an equity standpoint, she was hopeful that patients who live far from their transplant center or may face other difficulties in getting to appointments can now be more engaged with their providers. Purnell advocated for thinking of ways to continue to revolutionize the field, prioritizing building trust with patients and their caregivers, which could help to improve long-term outcomes.

Rosenbaum recounted the number of times throughout the workshop that speakers had highlighted the differences in immune responses among different ethnic groups, and asked how the transplant medical community accounts for those differences in planning for both the procedure and recovery. Are differences tracked separately in studies looking at transplant outcomes? Purnell replied by highlighting the variability among transplant center practices, so answers will often be different depending on setting. Most of what is known comes from the national registries, which include numerous types of information, but they all use standard risk adjustment models as well to control for certain factors.

FINAL THOUGHTS

Finally, Rosenbaum called for comments and reflections from speakers, wanting to ensure they were heard by SSA and the public. Lease commented that the discussions throughout the workshop highlighted the variety of issues many transplant patients face, many of which are nonmedical, such as accessing care or continuing strict adherence to difficult protocols. Gupta emphasized this concept as well, saying that each transplant recipient or candidate is different from the next, creating a need to target policy solutions to address the specific needs of individuals from different backgrounds. She called attention to the numerous barriers patients encounter when merely trying to get on the transplant list, so simplifying the process overall would be hugely beneficial. Tying in diversity, Gupta said many transplant patients do not trust the system because things are so complex, and they may have had negative experiences in the past—so she called for getting these patients more engaged and empowered to have more successful outcomes. Patel concluded, noting the need to address disincentives associated with disability and health care coverage. He explained that if transplant patients were to become more active and start to work, they might lose their health care coverage, which would threaten their access to critical immunosuppressive medications. While there has been progress on this front over the past few years, Patel acknowledged, such issues need to be addressed more directly.

References

AHA (American Heart Association). 2021. *The impact of congenital heart defects*. https://www.heart.org/en/health-topics/congenital-heart-defects/the-impact-of-congenital-heart-defects (accessed June 9, 2021).

Alraies, M. C., and P. Eckman. 2014. Adult heart transplant: Indications and outcomes. *Journal of Thoracic Disease* 6(8):1120–1128.

Andreoni, K. A., R. Forbes, R. M. Andreoni, G. Phillips, H. Stewart, and M. Ferris. 2013. Age-related kidney transplant outcomes: Health disparities amplified in adolescence. *JAMA Internal Medicine* 173(16):1524–1532.

Arriola, K. J. 2017. Race, racism, and access to renal transplantation among African Americans. *Journal of Health Care for the Poor and Underserved* 28(1):30–45.

Bachmann, J. M., A. S. Shah, M. S. Duncan, R. A. Greevy, Jr., A. J. Graves, S. Ni, H. H. Ooi, T. J. Wang, R. J. Thomas, M. A. Whooley, and M. S. Freiberg. 2018. Cardiac rehabilitation and readmissions after heart transplantation. *Journal of Heart and Lung Transplantation* 37(4):467–476.

Bae, S., A. B. Massie, X. Luo, S. Anjum, N. M. Desai, and D. L. Segev. 2016. Changes in discard rate after the introduction of the kidney donor profile index (KDPI). *American Journal of Transplantation* 16(7):2202–2207.

Bailey, Z. D., N. Krieger, M. Agénor, J. Graves, N. Linos, and M. T. Bassett. 2017. Structural racism and health inequities in the USA: Evidence and interventions. *The Lancet* 389(10077):1453–1463.

Bajwah, S., A. O. Oluyase, D. Yi, W. Gao, C. J. Evans, G. Grande, C. Todd, M. Costantini, F. E. Murtagh, and I. J. Higginson. 2020. The effectiveness and cost-effectiveness of hospital-based specialist palliative care for adults with advanced illness and their caregivers. *Cochrane Database of Systematic Reviews* 9:CD012780.

Barbot, O. 2014. *Baltimore City health disparities report card 2013.* https://health.baltimorecity.gov/sites/default/files/Health%20Disparities%20Report%20Card%20FINAL%2024-Apr-14.pdf (accessed June 9, 2021).

Berquist, R. K., W. E. Berquist, C. O. Esquivel, K. L. Cox, K. I. Wayman, and I. F. Litt. 2006. Adolescent non-adherence: Prevalence and consequences in liver transplant recipients. *Pediatric Transplantation* 10(3):304–310.

Boyarsky, B. J., W. A. Werbel, R. K. Avery, A. A. R. Tobian, A. B. Massie, D. L. Segev, and J. M. Garonzik-Wang. 2021. Immunogenicity of a single dose of SARS-CoV-2 messenger RNA vaccine in solid organ transplant recipients. *JAMA* 325(17):1784–1786.

Brito-Costa, A., L. Pereira-da-Silva, A. L. Papoila, M. Alves, É. Mateus, F. Nolasco, and E. Barroso. 2016. Factors associated with changes in body composition shortly after orthotopic liver transplantation: The potential influence of immunosuppressive agents. *Transplantation* 100(8):1714–1722.

Butler, C. R., P. P. Reese, J. D. Perkins, Y. N. Hall, J. R. Curtis, M. Kurella Tamura, and A. M. O'Hare. 2020. End-of-life care among us adults with eskd who were waitlisted or received a kidney transplant, 2005–2014. *Journal of the American Society of Nephrology* 31(10):2424–2433.

Castleberry, A., M. S. Mulvihill, B. A. Yerokun, B. C. Gulack, B. Englum, L. Snyder, M. Worni, A. Osho, S. Palmer, R. D. Davis, and M. G. Hartwig. 2017. The utility of 6-minute walk distance in predicting waitlist mortality for lung transplant candidates. *The Journal of heart and lung transplantation* 36(7):780–786.

CDC (Centers for Disease Control and Prevention). 2020a. *Heart disease facts.* https://www.cdc.gov/heartdisease/fcts.htm (accessed June 9, 2021).

CDC. 2020b. *Hepatitis C questions and answers for the public.* https://www.cdc.gov/hepatitis/hcv/cfaq.htm (accessed June 9, 2021).

CDC. 2021. *Chronic kidney disease in the United States.* Atlanta, GA: Centers for Disease Control and Prevention, U.S. Department of Health and Human Services.

Chambers, D. C., W. S. Cherikh, M. O. Harhay, D. Hayes, Jr., E. Hsich, K. K. Khush, B. Meiser, L. Potena, J. W. Rossano, A. E. Toll, T. P. Singh, A. Sadavarte, A. Zuckermann, J. Stehlik, and the International Society for Heart and Lung Transplantation. 2019. The International Thoracic Organ Transplant Registry of the International Society for Heart and Lung Transplantation: Thirty-sixth adult lung and heart-lung transplantation report-2019; focus theme: Donor and recipient size match. *The Journal of Heart and Lung Transplantation* 38(10):1042–1055.

Chang, C. F., R. P. Winsett, A. Osama Gaber, and D. K. Hathaway. 2004. Cost-effectiveness of post-transplantation quality of life intervention among kidney recipients. *Clinical Transplantation* 18(4):407–414.

Devine, J. F. 2008. Chronic obstructive pulmonary disease: An overview. *American Health & Drug Benefits* 1(7):34–42.

Dew, M. A., R. L. Kormos, A. F. DiMartini, G. E. Switzer, H. C. Schulberg, L. H. Roth, and B. P. Griffith. 2001. Prevalence and risk of depression and anxiety-related disorders during the first three years after heart transplantation. *Psychosomatics* 42(4):300–313.

Dew, M. A., E. M. Rosenberger, L. Myaskovsky, A. F. DiMartini, A. J. DeVito Dabbs, D. M. Posluszny, J. Steel, G. E. Switzer, D. A. Shellmer, and J. B. Greenhouse. 2015. Depression and anxiety as risk factors for morbidity and mortality after organ transplantation: A systematic review and meta-analysis. *Transplantation* 100(5):988–1003.

DiMartini, A., C. Crone, M. Fireman, and M. A. Dew. 2008. Psychiatric aspects of organ transplantation in critical care. *Critical Care Clinics* 24(4):949–981.

Dipchand, A. I., R. Kirk, L. B. Edwards, A. Y. Kucheryavaya, C. Benden, J. D. Christie, F. Dobbels, L. H. Lund, A. O. Rahmel, R. D. Yusen, and J. Stehlik. 2013. The registry of the International Society for Heart and Lung Transplantation: Sixteenth official pediatric heart transplantation report—2013; focus theme: Age. *The Journal of Heart and Lung Transplantation* 32(10):979–988.

Ekong, U. D., N. A. Gupta, R. Urban, and W. S. Andrews. 2019. 20- to 25-year patient and graft survival following a single pediatric liver transplant-analysis of the United Network of Organ Sharing database: Where to go from here. *Pediatric Transplantation* 23(6):e13523.

Engle, D. 2001. Psychosocial aspects of the organ transplant experience: What has been established and what we need for the future. *Journal of Clinical Psychology* 57(4):521–549.

Exterkate, L., B. R. Slegtenhorst, M. Kelm, M. Seyda, J. M. Schuitenmaker, M. Quante, H. Uehara, A. El Khal, and S. G. Tullius. 2016. Frailty and transplantation. *Transplantation* 100(4):727–733.

Ferris, M. E., D. S. Gipson, P. L. Kimmel, and P. W. Eggers. 2006. Trends in treatment and outcomes of survival of adolescents initiating end-stage renal disease care in the United States of America. *Pediatric Nephrology* 21(7):1020–1026.

Florian, J., A. Rubin, R. Mattiello, F. F. Fontoura, J. Camargo Jde, and P. J. Teixeira. 2013. Impact of pulmonary rehabilitation on quality of life and functional capacity in patients on waiting lists for lung transplantation. *Jornal Brasileiro de Pneumologia* 39(3):349–356.

Fredericks, E. M., M. J. Lopez, J. C. Magee, V. Shieck, and L. Opipari-Arrigan. 2007. Psychological functioning, nonadherence and health outcomes after pediatric liver transplantation. *American Journal of Transplantation* 7(8):1974–1983.

Fried, L. P., C. M. Tangen, J. Walston, A. B. Newman, C. Hirsch, J. Gottdiener, T. Seeman, R. Tracy, W. J. Kop, G. Burke, and M. A. McBurnie. 2001. Frailty in older adults: Evidence for a phenotype. *The Journal of Gerontology, Series A: Biological Sciences and Medical Sciences* 56(3):M146–M156.

Fuller, L. M., B. Button, B. Tarrant, C. R. Battistuzzo, M. Braithwaite, G. Snell, and A. E. Holland. 2014. Patients' expectations and experiences of rehabilitation following lung transplantation. *Clinical Transplantation* 28(2):252–258.

Garonzik-Wang, J. M., P. Govindan, J. W. Grinnan, M. Liu, H. M. Ali, A. Chakraborty, V. Jain, R. L. Ros, N. T. James, L. M. Kucirka, E. C. Hall, J. C. Berger, R. A. Montgomery, N. M. Desai, N. N. Dagher, C. J. Sonnenday, M. J. Englesbe, M. A. Makary, J. D. Walston, and D. L. Segev. 2012. Frailty and delayed graft function in kidney transplant recipients. *Archives of Surgery* 147(2):190–193.

Gogtay, N., J. N. Giedd, L. Lusk, K. M. Hayashi, D. Greenstein, A. C. Vaituzis, T. F. Nugent, 3rd, D. H. Herman, L. S. Clasen, A. W. Toga, J. L. Rapoport, and P. M. Thompson. 2004. Dynamic mapping of human cortical development during childhood through early adulthood. *Proceedings of the National Academy of Sciences* 101(21):8174–8179.

Gonzalez-Jaramillo, V., V. Fuhrer, N. Gonzalez-Jaramillo, D. Kopp-Heim, S. Eychmüller, and M. Maessen. 2020. Impact of home-based palliative care on health care costs and hospital use: A systematic review. *Palliat Support Care* 1–14.

Goodman, D. M., M. Hall, A. Levin, R. S. Watson, R. G. Williams, S. S. Shah, and A. D. Slonim. 2011. Adults with chronic health conditions originating in childhood: Inpatient experience in children's hospitals. *Pediatrics* 128(1):5–13.

Grady, K. L., D. C. Naftel, J. B. Young, D. Pelegrin, J. Czerr, R. Higgins, A. Heroux, B. Rybarczyk, M. McLeod, J. Kobashigawa, J. Chait, C. White-Williams, S. Myers, and J. K. Kirklin. 2007. Patterns and predictors of physical functional disability at 5 to 10 years after heart transplantation. *Journal of Heart and Lung Transplantation* 26(11):1182–1191.

Gupta, A., J. D. Mahnken, D. K. Johnson, T. S. Thomas, D. Subramaniam, T. Polshak, I. Gani, G. John Chen, J. M. Burns, and M. J. Sarnak. 2017. Prevalence and correlates of cognitive impairment in kidney transplant recipients. *BMC Nephrology* 18(1):158.

Gupta, A., T. S. Thomas, J. A. Klein, R. N. Montgomery, J. D. Mahnken, D. K. Johnson, D. A. Drew, M. J. Sarnak, and J. M. Burns. 2018. Discrepancies between perceived and measured cognition in kidney transplant recipients: Implications for clinical management. *Nephron* 138(1):22–28.

Gupta, A., R. N. Montgomery, V. Bedros, J. Lesko, J. D. Mahnken, S. Chakraborty, D. Drew, J. A. Klein, T. S. Thomas, A. Ilahe, P. Budhiraja, W. M. Brooks, T. M. Schmitt, M. J. Sarnak, J. M. Burns, and D. M. Cibrik. 2019. Subclinical cognitive impairment and listing for kidney transplantation. *Clinical Journal of the American Society of Nephrology* 14(4):567–575.

Gustafson, C., and M. K. Song. 2020. State of the science of palliative care in solid organ transplantation. *Progress in Transplantation* 30(4):382–395.

Haugen, C. E., A. Mountford, F. Warsame, R. Berkowitz, S. Bae, A. G. Thomas, C. H. Brown, D. C. Brennan, K. J. Neufeld, M. C. Carlson, D. L. Segev, M. McAdams-DeMarco. 2018. Incidence, risk factors, and sequelae of post-kidney transplant delirium. *Journal of the American Society of Nephrology* 2018010064.

Haugen, C. E., N. M. Chu, H. Ying, F. Warsame, C. M. Holscher, N. M. Desai, M. R. Jones, S. P. Norman, D. C. Brennan, J. Garonzik-Wang, J. D. Walston, A. W. Bingaman, D. L. Segev, and M. McAdams-DeMarco. 2019. Frailty and access to kidney transplantation. *Clinical Journal of the American Society of Nephrology* 14(4):576–582.

Hayanga, J. W. A., H. K. Hayanga, S. D. Holmes, Y. Ren, N. Shigemura, V. Badhwar, and G. Abbas. 2019. Mechanical ventilation and extracorporeal membrane oxygenation as a bridge to lung transplantation: Closing the gap. *The Journal of Heart and Lung Transplantation* 38(10):1104–1111.

Hayes, D., Jr., W. S. Cherikh, D. C. Chambers, M. O. Harhay, K. K. Khush, R. R. Lehman, B. Meiser, J. W. Rossano, E. Hsich, L. Potena, A. Sadavarte, T. P. Singh, A. Zuckermann, J. Stehlik, and the International Society for Heart and Lung Transplatation. 2019. The International Thoracic Organ Transplant Registry of the International Society for Heart and Lung Transplantation: Twenty-second pediatric lung and heart-lung transplantation report 2019; focus theme: Donor and recipient size match. *The Journal of Heart and Lung Transplantation* 38(10):1015–1027.

Horslen, S. P., J. M. Smith, Y. Ahn, M. A. Skeans, M. Cafarella, S. M. Noreen, J. J. Snyder, and A. K. Israni. 2021. OPTN/SRTR 2019 annual data report: Intestine. *American Journal of Transplantation* 21(S2):316–355.

Janaudis-Ferreira, T., C. M. Tansey, S. Mathur, T. Blydt-Hansen, J. Lamoureaux, A. Rakel, N. P. de Sousa Maia, A. Bussieres, S. Ahmed, and J. Boruff. 2021. The effects of exercise training in adult solid organ transplant recipients: A systematic review and meta-analysis. *Transplant International* 34(5):801–824.

Johnson, M. A. J., K. Javalkar, M. van Tilburg, C. Haberman, E. Rak, and M. E. Ferris. 2015. The relationship of transition readiness, self-efficacy, and adherence to preferred health learning method by youths with chronic conditions. *Journal of Pediatric Nursing* 30(5):e83–e90.

Karnofsky, D. A., W. H. Abelmann, L. F. Craver, and J. H. Burchenal. 1948. The use of the nitrogen mustards in the palliative treatment of carcinoma. With particular reference to bronchogenic carcinoma. *Cancer* 1(4):634–656.

Katz, M., S. Gillespie, J. P. Stevens, L. Hall, V. Kolachala, R. Ford, K. Levin, and N. A. Gupta. 2021. African american pediatric liver transplant recipients have an increased risk of death after transferring to adult healthcare. *The Journal of Pediatrics* 233:119–125.

Khush, K. K., W. S. Cherikh, D. C. Chambers, M. O. Harhay, D. Hayes, Jr., E. Hsich, B. Meiser, L. Potena, A. Robinson, J. W. Rossano, A. Sadavarte, T. P. Singh, A. Zuckermann, and J. Stehlik. 2019. The International Thoracic Organ Transplant Registry of the International Society for Heart and Lung Transplantation: Thirty-sixth adult heart transplantation report; focus theme: Donor and recipient size match. *The Journal of Heart and Lung Transplantation* 38(10):1056–1066.

Kobashigawa, J. A., D. A. Leaf, N. Lee, M. P. Gleeson, H. Liu, M. A. Hamilton, J. D. Moriguchi, N. Kawata, K. Einhorn, E. Herlihy, and H. Laks. 1999. A controlled trial of exercise rehabilitation after heart transplantation. *New England Journal of Medicine* 340(4):272–277.

Kobashigawa, J., D. Dadhania, S. Bhorade, D. Adey, J. Berger, G. Bhat, M. Budev, A. Duarte-Rojo, M. Dunn, S. Hall, M. N. Harhay, K. L. Johansen, S. Joseph, C. C. Kennedy, E. Kransdorf, K. L. Lentine, R. J. Lynch, M. McAdams-DeMarco, S. Nagai, M. Olymbios, J. Patel, S. Pinney, J. Schaenman, D. L. Segev, P. Shah, L. G. Singer, J. P. Singer, C. Sonnenday, P. Tandon, E. Tapper, S. G. Tullius, M. Wilson, M. Zamora, and J. C. Lai. 2019. Report from the American Society of Transplantation on frailty in solid organ transplantation. *American Journal of Transplantation* 19(4):984–994.

Kwong, A., W. R. Kim, J. R. Lake, J. M. Smith, D. P. Schladt, M. A. Skeans, S. M. Noreen, J. Foutz, E. Miller, J. J. Snyder, A. K. Israni, and B. L. Kasiske. 2020. OPTN/SRTR 2018 annual data report: Liver. *American Journal of Transplantation* 20(S1):193–299.

Kwong, A. J., W. R. Kim, J. R. Lake, J. M. Smith, D. P. Schladt, M. A. Skeans, S. M. Noreen, J. Foutz, S. E. Booker, M. Cafarella, J. J. Snyder, A. K. Israni, and B. L. Kasiske. 2021. OPTN/SRTR 2019 annual data report: Liver. *American Journal of Transplantation* 21(S2):208–315.

Lai, J. C., J. L. Dodge, M. R. Kappus, R. Wong, Y. Mohamad, D. L. Segev, and M. McAdams-DeMarco. 2021. A multicenter pilot randomized clinical trial of a home-based exercise program for patients with cirrhosis: The strength training intervention (strive). *The American Journal of Gastroenterology* 116(4):717–722.

Langer, D. 2015. Rehabilitation in patients before and after lung transplantation. *Respiration* 89(5):353–362.

Langone, A. J., L. Chan, P. Bolin, and M. Cooper. 2011. Enteric-coated mycophenolate sodium versus mycophenolate mofetil in renal transplant recipients experiencing gastrointestinal intolerance: A multicenter, double-blind, randomized study. *Transplantation* 91(4):470–478.

Lansky, S. B., M. A. List, L. L. Lansky, C. Ritter-Sterr, and D. R. Miller. 1987. The measurement of performance in childhood cancer patients. *Cancer* 60(7):1651–1656.

Lepping, R. J., R. N. Montgomery, P. Sharma, J. D. Mahnken, E. D. Vidoni, I.-Y. Choi, M. J. Sarnak, W. M. Brooks, J. M. Burns, and A. Gupta. 2021. Normalization of cerebral blood flow, neurochemicals, and white matter integrity after kidney transplantation. *Journal of the American Society of Nephrology* 32(1):177.

Li, M., S. Mathur, N. A. Chowdhury, D. Helm, and L. G. Singer. 2013. Pulmonary rehabilitation in lung transplant candidates. *Journal of Heart and Lung Transplantation* 32(6):626–632.

Markell, M. S., A. DiBenedetto, V. Maursky, N. Sumrani, J. H. Hong, D. A. Distant, A. M. Miles, B. G. Sommer, and E. A. Friedman. 1997. Unemployment in inner-city renal transplant recipients: Predictive and sociodemographic factors. *American Journal of Kidney Diseases* 29(6):881–887.

Massierer, D., N. Bourgeois, A. Räkel, K. Prévost, L. C. Lands, C. Poirier, and T. Janaudis-Ferreira. 2020. Changes in 6-minute walking distance in lung transplant candidates while participating in a home-based pre-habilitation program—a retrospective chart review. *Clinical Transplantation* 34(10):e14045.

McAdams-DeMarco, M. A., A. Law, M. L. Salter, B. Boyarsky, L. Gimenez, B. G. Jaar, J. D. Walston, and D. L. Segev. 2013a. Frailty as a novel predictor of mortality and hospitalization in individuals of all ages undergoing hemodialysis. *Journal of the American Geriatrics Society* 61(6):896–901.

McAdams-DeMarco, M. A., A. Law, M. L. Salter, E. Chow, M. Grams, J. Walston, and D. L. Segev. 2013b. Frailty and early hospital readmission after kidney transplantation. *American Journal of Transplantation* 13(8):2091–2095.

McAdams-DeMarco, M. A., A. Law, E. King, B. Orandi, M. Salter, N. Gupta, E. Chow, N. Alachkar, N. Desai, R. Varadhan, J. Walston, and D. L. Segev. 2015. Frailty and mortality in kidney transplant recipients. *American Journal of Transplantation* 15(1):149–154.

McAdams-DeMarco, M. A., E. A. King, X. Luo, C. Haugen, S. DiBrito, A. Shaffer, L. M. Kucirka, N. M. Desai, N. N. Dagher, B. E. Lonze, R. A. Montgomery, J. Walston, and D. L. Segev. 2017. Frailty, length of stay, and mortality in kidney transplant recipients: A national registry and prospective cohort study. *Annals of Surgery* 266(6):1084–1090.

McAdams-DeMarco, M. A., H. Ying, S. Van Pilsum Rasmussen, J. Schrack, C. E. Haugen, N. M. Chu, M. González Fernández, N. Desai, J. D. Walston, and D. L. Segev. 2019. Prehabilitation prior to kidney transplantation: Results from a pilot study. *Clinical Transplantation* 33(1):e13450.

McManus, M. A., L. R. Pollack, W. C. Cooley, J. W. McAllister, D. Lotstein, B. Strickland, and M. Y. Mann. 2013. Current status of transition preparation among youth with special needs in the United States. *Pediatrics* 131(6):1090–1097.

Meister, N. D., M. J. McAleer, J. S. Meister, J. E. Riley, and J. G. Copeland. 1986. Returning to work after heart transplantation. *Journal of Heart Transplantation* 5(2):154–161.

Morris, A. A., E. P. Kransdorf, B. L. Coleman, and M. Colvin. 2016. Racial and ethnic disparities in outcomes after heart transplantation: A systematic review of contributing factors and future directions to close the outcomes gap. *Journal of Heart and Lung Transplantation* 35(8):953–961.

Murray, A. M., D. E. Tupper, D. S. Knopman, D. T. Gilbertson, S. L. Pederson, S. Li, G. E. Smith, A. K. Hochhalter, A. J. Collins, and R. L. Kane. 2006. Cognitive impairment in hemodialysis patients is common. *Neurology* 67(2):216–223.

Newton, S. E. 2003. Relationship between depression and work outcomes following liver transplantation: The nursing perspective. *Gastroenterology Nursing* 26(2):68–72.

Ng, V. L., E. M. Alonso, J. C. Bucuvalas, G. Cohen, C. A. Limbers, J. W. Varni, G. Mazariegos, J. Magee, S. V. McDiarmid, and R. Anand. 2012. Health status of children alive 10 years after pediatric liver transplantation performed in the US and Canada: Report of the studies of pediatric liver transplantation experience. *Journal of Pediatrics* 160(5):820–826.

Ohnemus, D., K. Neighbors, K. Rychlik, R. S. Venick, J. C. Bucuvalas, S. S. Sundaram, V. L. Ng, W. S. Andrews, Y. Turmelle, G. V. Mazariegos, L. G. Sorensen, and E. M. Alonso. 2020. Health-related quality of life and cognitive functioning in pediatric liver transplant recipients. *Liver Transplantation* 26(1):45–56.

OPTN (Organ Procurement and Transplantation Network). 2020a. *A guide to calculating and interpreting the estimated post-transplant survival (EPTS) score used in the kidney allocation system (KAS)*. https://optn.transplant.hrsa.gov/media/1511/guide_to_calculating_interpreting_epts.pdf (accessed June 9, 2021).

OPTN. 2020b. *A guide to calculating and interpreting the kidney donor profile index (KDPI)*. https://optn.transplant.hrsa.gov/media/1512/guide_to_calculating_interpreting_kdpi.pdf (accessed June 9, 2021).

Pantilat, S. Z., D. L. O'Riordan, S. L. Dibble, and C. S. Landefeld. 2012. Longitudinal assessment of symptom severity among hospitalized elders diagnosed with cancer, heart failure, and chronic obstructive pulmonary disease. *Journal of Hospital Medicine* 7(7):567–572.

Paraskeva, M. A., L. B. Edwards, B. Levvey, J. Stehlik, S. Goldfarb, R. D. Yusen, G. P. Westall, and G. I. Snell. 2018. Outcomes of adolescent recipients after lung transplantation: An analysis of the International Society for Heart and Lung Transplantation registry. *The Journal of Heart and Lung Transplantation* 37(3):323–331.

Paris, W., A. Woodbury, S. Thompson, M. Levick, S. Nothegger, P. Arbuckle, L. Hutkin-Slade, and D. K. Cooper. 1993. Returning to work after heart transplantation. *Journal of Heart and Lung Transplantation* 12(1 Pt 1):46–53; discussion 53–54.

Pflugrad, H., P. Nösel, X. Ding, B. Schmitz, H. Lanfermann, H. Barg-Hock, J. Klempnauer, M. Schiffer, and K. Weissenborn. 2020. Brain function and metabolism in patients with long-term tacrolimus therapy after kidney transplantation in comparison to patients after liver transplantation. *PLOS ONE* 15(3):e0229759.

Popel, J., R. Joffe, B. V. Acton, G. Y. Bond, A. R. Joffe, J. Midgley, C. M. T. Robertson, R. S. Sauve, and C. J. Morgan. 2019. Neurocognitive and functional outcomes at 5 years of age after renal transplant in early childhood. *Pediatric Nephrology* 34(5):889–895.

Porter, M. E. 2010. What is value in health care? *New England Journal of Medicine* 363(26):2477–2481.

Purnell, T. S., P. Auguste, D. C. Crews, J. Lamprea-Montealegre, T. Olufade, R. Greer, P. Ephraim, J. Sheu, D. Kostecki, N. R. Powe, H. Rabb, B. Jaar, and L. E. Boulware. 2013. Comparison of life participation activities among adults treated by hemodialysis, peritoneal dialysis, and kidney transplantation: A systematic review. *American Journal of Kidney Diseases* 62(5):953–973.

Purnell, T. S., E. A. Calhoun, S. H. Golden, J. R. Halladay, J. L. Krok-Schoen, B. M. Appelhans, and L. A. Cooper. 2016a. Achieving health equity: Closing the gaps in health care disparities, interventions, and research. *Health Affairs* 35(8):1410–1415.

Purnell, T. S., X. Luo, L. M. Kucirka, L. A. Cooper, D. C. Crews, A. B. Massie, L. E. Boulware, and D. L. Segev. 2016b. Reduced racial disparity in kidney transplant outcomes in the United States from 1990 to 2012. *Journal of the American Society of Nephrology* 27(8):2511–2518.

Purnell, T. S., X. Luo, D. C. Crews, S. Bae, J. M. Ruck, L. A. Cooper, M. E. Grams, M. L. Henderson, M. M. Waldram, M. Johnson, and D. L. Segev. 2019. Neighborhood poverty and sex differences in live donor kidney transplant outcomes in the United States. *Transplantation* 103(10):2183–2189.

Quinn, K. L., T. Stukel, N. M. Stall, A. Huang, S. Isenberg, P. Tanuseputro, R. Goldman, P. Cram, D. Kavalieratos, A. S. Detsky, and C. M. Bell. 2020. Association between palliative care and healthcare outcomes among adults with terminal non-cancer illness: Population based matched cohort study. *BMJ* 370:m2257.

Randall, H. B., T. Alhamad, M. A. Schnitzler, Z. Zhang, S. Ford-Glanton, D. A. Axelrod, D. L. Segev, B. L. Kasiske, G. P. Hess, H. Yuan, R. Ouseph, and K. L. Lentine. 2017. Survival implications of opioid use before and after liver transplantation. *Liver Transplantation* 23(3):305–314.

Rogal, S. S., M. A. Dew, P. Fontes, and A. F. DiMartini. 2013. Early treatment of depressive symptoms and long-term survival after liver transplantation. *American Journal of Transplantation* 13(4):928–935.

Rogal, S. S., K. Bielefeldt, A. D. Wasan, F. E. Lotrich, S. Zickmund, E. Szigethy, and A. F. DiMartini. 2015. Inflammation, psychiatric symptoms, and opioid use are associated with pain and disability in patients with cirrhosis. *Clinical Gastroenterology and Hepatology* 13(5):1009–1016.

Rosen, D. S., R. W. Blum, M. Britto, S. M. Sawyer, and D. M. Siegel. 2003. Transition to adult health care for adolescents and young adults with chronic conditions: Position paper of the society for adolescent medicine. *Journal of Adolescent Health* 33(4):309–311.

Rossano, J. W., T. P. Singh, W. S. Cherikh, D. C. Chambers, M. O. Harhay, D. Hayes, Jr., E. Hsich, K. K. Khush, B. Meiser, L. Potena, A. E. Toll, A. Sadavarte, A. Zuckermann, J. Stehlik, and the International Society for Heart and Lung Transplantation. 2019. The International Thoracic Organ Transplant Registry of the International Society for Heart and Lung Transplantation: Twenty-second pediatric heart transplantation report 2019; focus theme: Donor and recipient size match. *The Journal of Heart and Lung Transplantation* 38(10):1028–1041.

Ruppert, K., S. Kuo, A. DiMartini, and V. Balan. 2010. In a 12-year study, sustainability of quality of life benefits after liver transplantation varies with pretransplantation diagnosis. *Gastroenterology* 139(5):1619–1629.

Schoenherr, L. A., K. E. Bischoff, A. K. Marks, D. L. O'Riordan, and S. Z. Pantilat. 2019. Trends in hospital-based specialty palliative care in the United States from 2013 to 2017. *JAMA Network Open* 2(12):e1917043.

Schoo, E., T. Gustaw, C. Barbalinardo, N. Rodrigues, Y. Zameni, S. Mathur, and T. Janaudis-Ferreira. 2017. Solid organ transplant recipients' opinions of pre- and posttransplant supervised exercise programmes: A brief report. *Physiotherapie Canada* 69(2):178–183.

Shemesh, E., R. A. Annunziato, R. Yehuda, B. L. Shneider, J. H. Newcorn, C. Hutson, J. A. Cohen, J. Briere, J. M. Gorman, and S. Emre. 2007. Childhood abuse, nonadherence, and medical outcome in pediatric liver transplant recipients. *Journal of the American Academy of Child and Adolescent Psychiatry* 46(10):1280–1289.

Shemesh, E., J. C. Bucuvalas, R. Anand, G. V. Mazariegos, E. M. Alonso, R. S. Venick, M. Reyes-Mugica, R. A. Annunziato, and B. L. Shneider. 2017. The medication level variability index (MLVI) predicts poor liver transplant outcomes: A prospective multi-site study. *American Journal of Transplantation* 17(10):2668–2678.

Siegel, R. L., K. D. Miller, and A. Jemal. 2018. Cancer statistics, 2018. *CA: A Cancer Journal for Clinicians* 68(1):7–30.

Squires, R. H., V. Ng, R. Romero, U. Ekong, W. Hardikar, S. Emre, and G. V. Mazariegos. 2014. Evaluation of the pediatric patient for liver transplantation: 2014 practice guideline by the American Association for the Study of Liver Diseases, American Society of Transplantation, and the North American Society for Pediatric Gastroenterology, Hepatology and Nutrition. *Hepatology* 60(1):362–398.

SRTR (Scientific Registry of Transplant Recipients). 2018. *OPTN/SRTR 2018 annual data report: Kidney*. https://srtr.transplant.hrsa.gov/annual_reports/2018/Kidney.aspx (accessed May 13, 2021).

Temel, J. S., J. A. Greer, A. Muzikansky, E. R. Gallagher, S. Admane, V. A. Jackson, C. M. Dahlin, C. D. Blinderman, J. Jacobsen, W. F. Pirl, J. A. Billings, and T. J. Lynch. 2010. Early palliative care for patients with metastatic non–small-cell lung cancer. *New England Journal of Medicine* 363(8):733–742.

Thomas, A. G., J. M. Ruck, N. M. Chu, D. Agoons, A. A. Shaffer, C. E. Haugen, B. Swenor, S. P. Norman, J. Garonzik-Wang, D. L. Segev, and M. McAdams-DeMarco. 2020. Kidney transplant outcomes in recipients with visual, hearing, physical and walking impairments: A prospective cohort study. *Nephrology, Dialysis, Transplantation* 35(7):1262–1270.

Toomey, S. L., A. T. Chien, M. N. Elliott, J. Ratner, and M. A. Schuster. 2013. Disparities in unmet need for care coordination: The national survey of children's health. *Pediatrics* 131(2):217–224.

Urschel, S., G. Y. Bond, I. A. Dinu, F. Moradi, J. Conway, G. Garcia-Guerra, B. V. Acton, A. R. Joffe, M. AlAklabi, I. M. Rebeyka, and C. M. T. Robertson. 2018. Neurocognitive outcomes after heart transplantation in early childhood. *Journal of Heart and Lung Transplantation* 37(6):740–748.

Valapour, M., C. J. Lehr, M. A. Skeans, J. M. Smith, E. Miller, R. Goff, J. Foutz, A. K. Israni, J. J. Snyder, and B. L. Kasiske. 2021. OPTN/SRTR 2019 annual data report: Lung. *American Journal of Transplantation* 21(S2):441–520.

Van Arendonk, K. J., N. T. James, B. J. Boyarsky, J. M. Garonzik-Wang, B. J. Orandi, J. C. Magee, J. M. Smith, P. M. Colombani, and D. L. Segev. 2013. Age at graft loss after pediatric kidney transplantation: Exploring the high-risk age window. *Clinical Journal of the American Society of Nephrology* 8(6):1019–1026.

Vieux, L., A. A. Simcox, Z. Mediouni, P. Wild, M. Koller, R. K. Studer, and B. Danuser. 2019. Predictors of return to work 12 months after solid organ transplantation: Results from the Swiss Transplant Cohort study. *Journal of Occupational Rehabilitation* 29(2):462–471.

Virani, S. S., A. Alonso, E. J. Benjamin, M. S. Bittencourt, C. W. Callaway, A. P. Carson, A. M. Chamberlain, A. R. Chang, S. Cheng, F. N. Delling, L. Djousse, M. S. V. Elkind, J. F. Ferguson, M. Fornage, S. S. Khan, B. M. Kissela, K. L. Knutson, T. W. Kwan, D. T. Lackland, T. T. Lewis, J. H. Lichtman, C. T. Longenecker, M. S. Loop, P. L. Lutsey, S. S. Martin, K. Matsushita, A. E. Moran, M. E. Mussolino, A. M. Perak, W. D. Rosamond, G. A. Roth, U. K. A. Sampson, G. M. Satou, E. B. Schroeder, S. H. Shah, C. M. Shay, N. L. Spartano, A. Stokes, D. L. Tirschwell, L. B. VanWagner, and C. W. Tsao. 2020. Heart disease and stroke statistics—2020 update: A report from the American Heart Association. *Circulation* 141(9):e139–e596.

WHO (World Health Organization). 2020. *Palliative care.* https://www.who.int/news-room/fact-sheets/detail/palliative-care (accessed May 13, 2021).

Wong, R. J., and A. K. Singal. 2020. Trends in liver disease etiology among adults awaiting liver transplantation in the United States, 2014–2019. *JAMA Network Open* 3(2):e1920294.

Zhong, Y., D. B. Gilleskie, M. A. L. van Tilburg, S. R. Hooper, E. Rak, K. Javalkar, M. Nazareth, B. Pitts, M. Ndugga, N. Jain, L. Hart, S. Bhansali, J. Richards, R. K. Detwiler, K. True, A. S. F. de Pomposo, and M. E. Ferris. 2018. Longitudinal self-management and/or transition readiness per the Transition Index among patients with chronic conditions in pediatric or adult care settings. *The Journal of Pediatrics* 203:361–370.

Appendix A

Statement of Task

In response to a request from the U.S. Social Security Administration (SSA), a planning committee of the National Academies of Sciences, Engineering, and Medicine (the National Academies) will organize and host a 1.5-day public workshop that will examine disability associated with organ transplantation. In particular, the workshop will include presentations on the functional outcomes for individuals who are recipients of organ transplants, including those of the kidney, liver, and lung.

The workshop will feature invited presentations and panel discussions on topics that may include

- Processes conducted to identify transplant recipients with the highest probability of positive posttransplantation outcomes;
- Current outcome measures for assessing effectiveness of care for individuals who have received organ transplantation (e.g., morbidity and mortality);
- Treatments used to improve a person's physical or mental functioning following organ transplant, and the settings in which the treatments are provided;
- The typical length of time from transplant surgery until the person's functioning improves to the point of which the condition is no longer disabling, and specific ages or other recipient traits where improvement is more likely;

- Laboratory or other findings used to assess medical and functional improvement after organ transplant; and
- Recent medical advances or new technologies that may alter expected patient outcomes, and potential advances anticipated in the near future.

The planning committee will develop the agenda for the workshop sessions, select and invite speakers and discussants, and moderate the discussions. A proceedings of the presentations and discussions at the workshop will be prepared by a designated rapporteur in accordance with institutional guidelines.

Appendix B

Workshop Agenda

MARCH 22, 2021

12:30 p.m. **Welcome and Workshop Overview**
Sara Rosenbaum, The George Washington University
Workshop Planning Committee Chair

Sponsor Remarks from the U.S. Social Security Administration (SSA)
Gina P. Clemons, SSA
Vincent Nibali, SSA

12:50 p.m. **Session 1: Solid Organ Transplantation in the United States: Clinical Challenges for Organ Recipient Functioning**
Moderator: Paul Kimmel, National Institute of Diabetes and Digestive and Kidney Diseases (NIDDK), National Institutes of Health (NIH)

Overview and Current Trends of the Organ Transplantation System
- David Mulligan, Organ Procurement and Transplantation Network (OPTN)

Clinical Conditions, Organ Transplants, and the Consequences for Health and Function in Adults

Kidney Transplantation
- Dorry Segev, Johns Hopkins University (JHU)

Liver Transplantation
- Shari Rogal, University of Pittsburgh; VA Pittsburgh Healthcare System

Lung Transplantation
- Erika Lease, University of Washington

Heart Transplantation
- Hannah Valantine, Stanford University

Disparities in Transplantation Recovery and Survival
- Tanjala Purnell, JHU

Panel Discussion

2:30 p.m. **Break**

2:45 p.m. **Session 2: Transplantation Over the Life Course: Transplants in Children and Adolescents and the Consequences for Adulthood**
Moderators:
Paul Kimmel, NIDDK, NIH
Dorry Segev, JHU

Clinical Conditions, Organ Transplants, and the Consequences for Health and Function in Children

Kidney Transplantation
- Maria E. Diaz-Gonzalez de Ferris, University of North Carolina Children's Research Institute

Liver/Intestine Transplantation
- George V. Mazariegos, University of Pittsburgh Medical Center Children's Hospital of Pittsburgh

Lung Transplantation
- Carol Conrad, Lucile Packard Children's Hospital

Heart Transplantation
- Clifford Chin, Cincinnati Children's Hospital Medical Center

Adolescent Posttransplant Transitions to Adulthood
- Nitika Gupta, Emory University

Panel Discussion

4:00 p.m. Session 3: Experiences of Organ Recipients and Their Caregivers
Moderators:
Melissa McQueen, Transplant Families
Robert Montgomery, New York University Langone Transplant Institute

Social Worker Perspective
- Charlie Thomas, Banner-University Medical Center Phoenix

Caregiver Perspective
- Melissa McQueen, Transplant Families

Organ Recipient Perspective
- Valen Keefer
- Dawn Edwards
- Stephanie Hoyt-Trapp
- Fanny Vlahos
- Robert Montgomery

Panel Discussion

5:10 p.m.   **Closing Remarks**
            Paul Kimmel, NIDDK, NIH

5:15 p.m.   **Adjourn Day 1**

MARCH 23, 2021

10:00 a.m. **Welcome and Workshop Overview**
            Sara Rosenbaum, The George Washington University
            Workshop Planning Committee Chair

10:05 a.m. **Session 4: Treatments, Technologies, and Interventions Affecting Posttransplant Functioning**
            Moderators:
            Dorry Segev, JHU
            Hannah Valantine, Stanford University

            Pretransplant Care Management Approaches
            - Mara McAdams-DeMarco, JHU

            Pharmacologic Treatments in Transplantation
            - Saeed Mohammad, Northwestern University Feinberg School of Medicine

            Posttransplant Rehabilitation: Optimizing Long-Term Outcomes After Transplant
            - Sunita Mathur, University of Toronto

            Palliative Care in Solid Organ Transplantation
            - Kirsten Wentlandt, University Health Network, Toronto

            Panel Discussion

11:15 a.m. **Session 5A: Assessing Physical, Cognitive, and Psychosocial Function After Organ Transplantation in Adults**
            Moderators:
            Erika Lease, University of Washington
            Shari Rogal, University of Pittsburgh; VA Pittsburgh Healthcare System

Assessing Physical Functioning in Organ Transplantation
- Jignesh Patel, Cedars-Sinai Medical Center

Cognition in Organ Transplantation
- Aditi Gupta, University of Kansas Medical Center

Psychosocial and Emotional Functioning in Transplantation
- Andrea DiMartini, University of Pittsburgh

Panel Discussion

12:15 p.m. Break

12:30 p.m. **Session 5B: Assessing Physical, Cognitive, and Psychosocial Function After Organ Transplantation in Children**
Moderators:
Erika Lease, University of Washington
Shari Rogal, University of Pittsburgh; VA Pittsburgh Healthcare System

Physical and Cognitive Functioning in Pediatric Organ Transplantation
- Saeed Mohammad, Northwestern University Feinberg School of Medicine

Psychosocial Risk Factors Associated with Clinical Outcomes in Children
- Eyal Shemesh, Mount Sinai Kravis Children's Hospital

Panel Discussion

1:20 p.m. Break

1:30 p.m.	**Session 6: The Future Outlook for Organ Transplantation and Disability** Moderators: Sara Rosenbaum, The George Washington University James Bowman, Health Resources and Services Administration **Panel Discussion** Panelists: • Aditi Gupta, University of Kansas Medical Center • Erika Lease, University of Washington • Jignesh Patel, Cedars-Sinai California Medical Center • Tanjala Purnell, JHU
2:10 p.m.	**Concluding Remarks** Sara Rosenbaum, The George Washington University Workshop Planning Committee Chair
2:15 p.m.	**Adjourn**

Appendix C

Biographical Sketches of Workshop Planning Committee Members and Speakers[1]

PLANNING COMMITTEE

Sara Rosenbaum, J.D. (*Chair*) is the Harold and Jane Hirsh Professor of Health Law and Policy and the founding chair of the Department of Health Policy at the Milken Institute School of Public Health at The George Washington University. She also holds professorships in the Trachtenberg School of Public Policy & Public Administration and the Schools of Law and Medicine & Health Sciences. A graduate of Wesleyan University and the Boston University School of Law, Dr. Rosenbaum has devoted her career to issues of health justice for populations who are medically underserved as a result of race, poverty, disability, or cultural exclusion. An honored teacher and scholar, a highly popular speaker, and a widely read writer on many aspects of health law and policy, Dr. Rosenbaum has emphasized public engagement as a core element of her professional life, providing public service to 6 presidential administrations and 19 Congresses. She is best known for her work on national health reform, Medicaid and private insurance, Medicaid managed care, health care access for medically underserved communities and populations, and civil rights and health care. Dr. Rosenbaum's current research focuses on the transformation of Medicaid and its effects on poor populations and

---

[1] Planning committee members marked with an asterisk also served as speakers at the workshop.

communities. She also focuses on national health reform, Medicaid managed care, and community health centers, the largest primary health care system for medically underserved rural and urban populations. She is best known for her research into the impact of laws affecting health care access and coverage and the potential effects of major shifts in laws affecting low income and medically underserved populations.

James Bowman, M.D., M.S., FACS, has been a senior physician with the Division of Transplantation at the Health Resources and Services Administration in the U.S. Department of Health and Human Services since 2009. Dr. Bowman supports the division's leadership in its oversight of the nation's solid organ and blood stem cell transplant programs. He served as a senior medical officer with the Chronic Care Policy Group at the Centers for Medicare & Medicaid Services in support of Medicare payment policy for end-stage renal disease/dialysis units, inpatient rehab hospitals, skilled nursing facilities, home health agencies, hospital prospective payment systems, and the physician fee schedule. He has medical management experience with several national health insurers and was a transplant and general surgeon in the U.S. Air Force and civilian practice. Dr. Bowman is a fellow of the American College of Surgeons and participates with the American Society of Transplant Surgeons and the American Society for Transplantation and Cellular Therapy. He earned his M.D. from Virginia Commonwealth University and his M.S. in management from North Carolina State University. He trained in general surgery at Wright State University and abdominal transplant surgery at the University of Pittsburgh and the Children's Hospital of Pittsburgh.

John A. Goss, M.D., FACS, is a professor of surgery in the Michael E. DeBakey Department of Surgery at the Baylor College of Medicine and the chief of the Abdominal Transplantation Division. He specializes in adult and pediatric liver transplantation, hepatobiliary surgery, and surgical management of liver tumors. He is board certified by the American Board of Surgery and a fellow of the American College of Surgeons. After earning his M.D. from Creighton University, Dr. Goss completed his general surgical residency at the Washington University School of Medicine in St. Louis Surgical Program. He then completed a 2-year multi-organ transplant fellowship in the Division of Liver and Pancreas Transplantation at the University of California, Los Angeles, David Geffen School of Medicine. Dr. Goss has performed many surgical "firsts" in Houston, including the first split liver adult and pediatric transplants, adult living donor liver transplant, dual organ lung–liver transplant, and dual organ heart–liver transplant.

Paul L. Kimmel, M.D., MACP, FRCP, FASN, has made significant contributions in patient care, research, and service to professional organizations. He has been a faculty member in the Department of Medicine at The George Washington University since 1983 and was the director of the university's Division of Renal Diseases and Hypertension Medical Center from 2001 to 2006. Dr. Kimmel served as the director of education for the American Society of Nephrology (ASN) from 2006 to 2007 and joined the National Institute of Diabetes and Digestive and Kidney Diseases at the National Institutes of Health in 2008. He is currently the senior advisor to the director of the Division of Kidney, Urologic, and Hematologic Diseases, where he has managed programs in HIV-associated kidney disease, acute kidney injury, clinical genetics of kidney disease, kidney precision medicine, clinical outcomes of kidney organ donation by African Americans, and opioid use in dialysis patients. His research interests include sleep disorders, quality of life, and psychosocial issues (including depression, anxiety, and perception of social support) in end-stage kidney disease and chronic kidney disease patients. He is also interested in HIV-associated kidney diseases, long-term outcomes of acute kidney injury, perception of pain, and inflammatory and immunologic factors mediating outcomes of kidney failure. He recently fostered patient and community engagement in clinical research. He has published more than 300 papers and edited 2 editions of the textbook *Chronic Renal Disease*. Dr. Kimmel served on the editorial boards of *Blood Purification*, the *American Journal of Kidney Diseases*, the *Journal of the American Society of Nephrology*, and the *Clinical Journal of the American Society of Nephrology*. He was recently inducted as a fellow of the Royal College of Physicians in London and is a master of the American College of Physicians. He served as a board member and the president of the National Academy of Medicine in Washington, DC. He received the Belding H. Scribner M.D. Memorial award from ASN in 2019. Dr. Kimmel received his M.D. from the New York University Grossman School of Medicine and trained in internal medicine at Bellevue Hospital in New York City. He completed a fellowship in renal and electrolyte disorders at the Hospital of the University of Pennsylvania and remained a faculty member until joining The George Washington University.

Erika D. Lease, M.D., FCCP,* is the medical director of the University of Washington Lung Transplant Program and an associate professor of medicine within the Division of Pulmonary, Critical Care and Sleep Medicine at the University of Washington. Dr. Lease also specializes in infectious diseases relating to all solid organ transplant recipients and is an attending with the Solid Organ Transplant Infectious Disease program. Her research interests include lung transplant, solid organ transplant, and infectious diseases.

George V. Mazariegos, M.D., FACS, FAST,* is the chief of the Pediatric Transplantation Division at the University of Pittsburgh Medical Center Children's Hospital of Pittsburgh, the Hillman Center for Pediatric Transplantation, and the Thomas E. Starzl Transplantation Institute. He is a professor at the University of Pittsburgh in the Departments of Surgery, Anesthesiology, and Critical Care Medicine and holds the Jamie Lee Curtis Chair in Surgery and Critical Care. Dr. Mazariegos earned a bachelor's degree in medical science at Northwestern University in 1984 and graduated from medical school there. He completed residency training at Michigan State University and fellowship training at the University of Pittsburgh in 1993. Dr. Mazariegos has been involved in the academic field of transplantation surgery for more than 25 years and served as the past chair of the Society of Pediatric Liver Transplantation, the immediate past president of the Intestinal Rehabilitation and Transplant Association, a counselor for the International Pediatric Transplant Association, and the immediate past chair of the United Network for Organ Sharing/Organ Procurement and Transplantation Network pediatric committee. He is a member of the International Liver Transplantation Society, the Society of University Surgeons, and the American Surgical Association. Recently, Dr. Mazariegos and colleagues founded the Starzl Network for Excellence in Pediatric Transplantation (www.starzlnetwork.org), a consortium bringing innovation and technology partners together with patients, families, and transplant centers to transform outcomes in children. Dr. Mazariegos authored or co-authored more than 265 original articles, more than 230 abstracts, and 20 book chapters.

Melissa McQueen* is the executive director of Transplant Families and works with parents and caregivers of children listed for or already having received a lifesaving organ transplant to help guide them to support, education, and assistance to help them through that difficult time. Ms. McQueen believes that education and support bring hope and healing for families. She volunteers with the United Network for Organ Sharing/Organ Procurement and Transplantation Network in their Pediatric Committee and their Data Advisory Committee, where she helped co-author "What Every Parent Needs to Know." She was also selected as a leader with Quality Improvement Collaboratives at the ACTION Learning Network (pediatric cardiac quality improvement [QI], Cincinnati Children's Hospital) and Starzl Learning Network (pediatric liver QI, University of Pittsburgh Medical Center) to give input and help co-create materials for clinicians and families. She worked on the spearheading committee that helped Donate Life America create National Pediatric Transplant Week (the last week of every April). She is the charter chair of the Heart Center Family Advisory Council and Alumni Patient and Family Advisory Council at Phoenix Children's Hospital. Ms. McQueen is a trained developer/engineer who has worked at companies such as Honeywell—Aeronautics Division, APS, Wells Fargo, and Phoenix Children's Hospital. Most recently, she helped to develop "My journey with" applications, covering patient education from diabetes to transplant for the newly diagnosed. Ms. McQueen holds a bachelor's degree in computer information systems from DeVry University.

Shari S. Rogal, M.D., M.P.H.,[*] is an assistant professor of medicine and transplant surgery at the University of Pittsburgh and a core member of the Center for Health Equity Research and Promotion, VA Healthcare System in Pittsburgh, Pennsylvania. Dr. Rogal is a transplant hepatologist whose clinical research focuses on addressing the psychosocial contributions to quality of life and transplant outcomes. She identified an association between untreated depression and increased rejection and mortality. Depression is associated with pain, and both conditions are often suboptimally managed in transplant populations. Dr. Rogal is currently developing and implementing a program to increase evidence-based management of these symptoms in the peritransplant period. Dr. Rogal also works in implementation science more broadly and has developed novel methods to assess the contributions of implementation strategies to the quality and equity of care.

Dorry Segev, M.D., Ph.D.,[*] is the Marjory K. and Thomas Pozefsky Professor of Surgery and Epidemiology and the associate vice chair of surgery at Johns Hopkins University. He is the founder and the director of the Epidemiology Research Group in Organ Transplantation. Dr. Segev was the first to demonstrate the survival benefit of incompatible kidney transplantation across the United States and is responsible for the first HIV–HIV transplants in the United States. His National Institutes of Health (NIH)-funded research includes kidney exchange, desensitization, long-term donor risk, access to transplantation, and expanding transplantation, including HIV positive donors, geographic disparities, posttransplant outcomes, and the intersection between transplantation and gerontology. Dr. Segev focuses on novel statistical and mathematical methods to simulate medical data, analysis of large health care data sets, and outcomes research. Dr. Segev published nearly 500 peer-reviewed research articles and was recently awarded the American Society of Transplantation's Clinical Science Investigator Award. He is a current councilor of the American Society of Transplant Surgeons and the former chair of the American Transplant Congress. His work has directly influenced policy, including two congressional bills (the Charlie W. Norwood Living Organ Donation Act for kidney exchange and the HIV Organ Policy Equity [HOPE] Act for HIV–HIV transplants). Dr. Segev is most inspired by his role as a mentor, having mentored more than 100 graduate students, residents, and faculty, and he is the only general surgeon in the United States funded by an NIH/National Institute of Diabetes and Digestive and Kidney Diseases Mentoring Grant.

Hannah Valantine, M.B.B.S., MRCP, FACC,* received her M.B.B.S. degree (bachelor of medicine, bachelor of surgery; the United Kingdom's equivalent to an M.D.) from St. George's, University of London, in 1978. She moved to the University of Hong Kong Li Ka Shing Faculty of Medicine for specialty training in elective surgery before returning to the United Kingdom. She was awarded a diploma of membership by the Royal College of Physicians in 1981. In addition, she completed postgraduate training and numerous fellowships, serving as the senior house officer in cardiology at Royal Brompton Hospital and the registrar in cardiology and general medicine at Hammersmith Hospital. In 1985, Dr. Valantine moved to the United States for postdoctoral training in cardiology at Stanford University. In 1988, she received a Doctor of Science, Medicine, from the University of London. Dr. Valantine became a clinical assistant professor in the Division of Cardiovascular Medicine at Stanford University and rose through the academic ranks to a full professor of medicine in the Division of Cardiovascular Medicine and the director of Heart Transplant Program. She came to the National Heart, Lung, and Blood Institute in 2014 to continue her research while also serving as the first chief officer of scientific workforce diversity. Dr. Valantine has received numerous awards, including a Best Doctor in America honor in 2002. She has authored more than 160 primary research articles and reviews and previously served on the editorial boards of the journals *Graft* and *Ethnicity & Disease*. Dr. Valantine's past and current memberships include the American College of Cardiology, the American Society of Transplant Physicians, and the American Heart Association. She was the past president of the American Heart Association Western States Affiliates.

WORKSHOP SPEAKERS

Clifford Chin, M.D., is a professor of pediatrics and the medical director of the Advanced Cardiomyopathy Services and Pediatric Heart Transplant at the Cincinnati Children's Hospital Medical Center. He completed his pediatric training at the University of California, Davis, Medical Center and pediatric cardiology postdoctoral fellowship at Stanford University. His academic focus has been on outcomes after transplantation, including prevention of posttransplant morbidity. He has collaborated with many pediatric and adult heart transplant colleagues, nationally and internationally, and outside the field of cardiology, including professionals in immunology, infectious diseases, oncology, and nephrology. His collaborative works include peer-reviewed publications, university and National Institutes of Health–funded projects, and patient care initiatives.

Carol Conrad, M.D., joined the clinical faculty at Stanford Children's Health/Lucile Packard Children's Hospital in 1995. Her training in pediatric (and adult) lung transplant began informally in 2004, and she was named the director of the program in 2007. The program separated from the adult service in 2009 and is the only pediatric program on the west coast, west of Texas. The team performs three pediatric lung or heart–lung transplants per year, on average, to treat cystic fibrosis, pulmonary hypertension, and some congenital vascular malformations that lead to pulmonary hypertension. Dr. Conrad's center has participated in national multicenter clinical research projects under the aegis of the Clinical Trials in Organ Transplantation in Children funding mechanism of the National Institutes of Health to discover mechanisms of lung graft failure in children. Dr. Conrad served as the chair of the Pediatric Scientific Council of the International Society for Heart and Lung Transplantation from 2019 to 2020, which then, under a reorganization business plan, became the representative of the Pediatric Lung Transplant Professional Community to the Advanced Lung Failure and Transplant steering committee. Dr. Conrad attended the Charles R. Drew/University of California, Los Angeles, Medical Education Program (1985–1989) and did her residency at the Children's Hospital Los Angeles in pediatrics (1989–1992). Dr. Conrad was a postdoctoral fellow (July 1992–July 1995) in the division of Pediatric Pulmonary Medicine at the Johns Hopkins University School of Medicine.

Andrea DiMartini, M.D., is a professor of psychiatry and surgery at the Thomas E. Starzl Transplantation Institute at the University of Pittsburgh. She completed her medical school training at the University of Chicago Pritzker School of Medicine and her residency at the Western Psychiatric Hospital. She has nearly 30 years of clinical and research experience working with the solid organ transplant teams at the Thomas E. Starzl Transplantation Institute. She is considered an expert in transplant psychiatry and has written extensively and lectures both nationally and internationally on these issues. She has been awarded several National Institutes of Health grants to conduct longitudinal research on patients' mental health and behavioral outcomes following transplantation.

Dawn P. Edwards is a self-described "27-year chronic kidney disease (CKD) warrior." Ms. Edwards has experienced firsthand every renal replacement modality, including a kidney transplant and rejection. She is currently a nocturnal home hemodialysis patient. She has extensive insight into the needs of people with CKD, always keeping in mind that they need different things at different times in their lives. Ms. Edwards is dedicated to improving the quality of life of people with kidney disease and also a resource to her community, sharing her story and educating people about the relationships among hypertension, diabetes, and kidney disease, especially in underserved communities. Ms. Edwards has served the community for more than 25 years through the IPRO End-Stage Renal Disease (ESRD) Network program of New York as a communicator, mentor, and educator. She is on many kidney disease–related boards and reinvented herself by working as a patient advocate for Fresenius/NxStage and a wellness ambassador for the Rogosin Institute. Ms. Edwards is also the co-chairperson of the National Forum of ESRD Networks Kidney Patient Advisory Council, actively involved with the National Kidney Foundation and the American Association of Kidney Patients, a patient advisor for studies with the National Institutes of Health and the National Institute of Diabetes and Digestive and Kidney Diseases, and the chief executive officer of her own advocacy and education organization, the New York State CKD Champions, whose motto is to educate, encourage, and empower. She believes that faith, family, and education are the keys to her longevity and every day is an opportunity to thrive, not just survive. Ms. Edwards recently co-authored an article in the January 2021 issue of *Clinical Journal of the American Society of Nephrology* titled "Personal Experiences of Patients in the Interaction of Culture and Kidney Disease."

Aditi Gupta, M.D., is a nephrologist and a clinical investigator with the long-term goal of pursuing impactful patient-oriented research in vascular risk reduction and dementia. After her training in internal medicine and nephrology, she started her career on the clinical educator track with a focus on clinical care and education. Having trained in the same program, she had the opportunity to follow many patients over the years who struggle with cognitive impairment and report improvement in cognition after a kidney transplant. These clinical observations inspired her to change her career path and immerse herself in clinical research. Dr. Gupta crossed interdepartmental boundaries, developed multidisciplinary collaborations, and embarked on and successfully completed challenging out-of-the-box studies. She received pilot grant awards from the Kidney Institute at the University of Kansas Medical Center, the Frontiers Pilot and Collaborative Studies Funding 4 Program, and the Office of Scholarly, Academic, & Research Mentoring. These led to a National Institutes of Health (NIH) K23 award in 2017 to examine cognition and brain changes from before to after kidney transplant to elucidate mechanisms underlying cognitive impairment in kidney disease. She has presented several abstracts and recently published a manuscript on brain changes from before to after transplant in the *Journal of the American Society of Nephrology*, a leading nephrology journal. She has two other investigator-initiated studies evaluating changes in cerebral blood flow with calcineurin inhibitors to understand observations of decrease in cerebral blood flow after transplantation in the K23 study. She has several studies investigating the prevalence of cognitive impairment in kidney transplantation and its impact on transplant candidacy. To further her research goals and bring changes in the real world in actual clinics, she trained in implementation science. This knowledge led to the NIH R61/R33 award Remote Monitoring and Virtual Collaborative Care for Hypertension Control to Prevent Cognitive Decline, funded in 2020. In this pragmatic study, she is testing a new hypertension program to achieve goal blood pressure to prevent cognitive decline.

Nitika Gupta, M.D., DCH, DNB, MRCPH, is a triple board-certified pediatric gastroenterologist and transplant hepatologist in the Department of Pediatrics at the Emory University School of Medicine and Children's Healthcare of Atlanta. She did her pediatric residency, pediatric gastroenterology, and transplant hepatology fellowships at Emory University. Over the past 20 years, the focus of her work has been in liver diseases of children and liver transplantation. She conducts basic, clinical, and translational research in pediatric liver transplantation and immune-mediated liver disease, such as autoimmune hepatitis and primary sclerosing cholangitis. She has received several honors for her work and published well-cited articles. She has a special interest in the transition of pediatric to adult health care and was the founding director of the adolescent transition program for liver transplant recipients. She also established a joint clinic between the pediatric and adult health care systems, resulting in improved graft and patient survival after transition. She has a strong focus on connecting the bench to the bedside with the overall goal of developing strategies and treatment options to improve the quality of life of children with liver disease and liver transplant. As she is in the southeast, a significant proportion of her patients are from minority backgrounds, and her recent research has demonstrated that significant racial disparities exist in African American children with liver disease and liver transplant with high risk of mortality after transferring from pediatric to adult health care. She has developed new interventions and programs to help mitigate these risks, resulting in improved outcomes. She is a member of the Diversity, Equity, and Inclusion councils of Children's Healthcare of Atlanta and the Emory University School of Medicine. She is interested in education and has mentored several undergraduates, medical students, residents, and fellows for laboratory and clinical research. She also serves on the Emory senate overseeing the university's activities, which includes several schools. She is on the American Board of Medical Specialties stakeholder committee and was selected to serve on its Vision commission, which was charged with developing a roadmap for the future of board certification of U.S. diplomats.

Stephanie Hoyt-Trapp, Ph.D., is a clinical–community psychologist. She received a new liver about 6 years ago after being diagnosed with non-alcoholic steatohepatitis. Severe depression and ongoing medical complications have made her transplant journey quite difficult. She faced portal hypertension, internal bleeding, encephalopathy, and an occluded hepatic vein. Dr. Hoyt-Trapp is currently working part time as a consulting psychologist on a grant regarding pain and cirrhosis.

Valen Keefer walks the line every day between survival and advocacy. At 38, she is thriving thanks to two lifesaving transplants resulting from polycystic kidney disease (PKD): a kidney when she was 19 and a liver at 35. Ms. Keefer has endured an arduous health journey full of hospital stays and illness. She has undergone 30 surgeries and has more than 60 inches of scars crisscrossing her body. Despite life challenging her at nearly every turn, Ms. Keefer is determined to help others who are fated to walk a similar path and hopes to be the role model she wishes she had. She has taken her new lease on life and is intent on paying it back 10-fold. As a passionate patient advocate since 2004, she works tirelessly to raise awareness of kidney disease, PKD, and organ donation and to help educate and empower others. Grounded in gratitude, Ms. Keefer works directly with countless patients and has shared her extraordinary story at more than 100 events across North America with an authentic optimism that inspires people and moves them to action. She has done many press interviews, coordinated educational and fundraising events, and helped raise more than $1 million for PKD research. Ms. Keefer has written hundreds of blogs (published by nonprofits), painting a genuine picture of the challenges and joys of this journey. Through her collaborations with numerous organizations, she has inspired 1.7 million social media followers with her story of hope and resilience that transforms people forever. Ms. Keefer has a way of connecting and touching the hearts and minds of all she meets, and her journey has become a beacon of hope for countless people around the world. She proves there is not just life post-transplant and with severe kidney disease but potentially a great one.

Sunita Mathur, B.Sc.P.T., Ph.D., is a physical therapist and an associate professor in the Department of Physical Therapy at the University of Toronto. She directs the Muscle Function and Performance Lab and conducts research on skeletal muscle dysfunction and sarcopenia in people with chronic lung disease and solid organ transplant candidates and recipients. The goals of the research program are to understand the link between muscle structure and function, the relationship between sarcopenia and clinical outcomes, and the effect of exercise training on improving muscle dysfunction. Dr. Mathur has published more than 100 peer-reviewed articles and holds grant funding from the Canadian Institutes of Health Research, Lung Health Foundation, and Canadian Thoracic Society. Dr. Mathur is the co-founder and the co-chair of the Canadian Network for Rehabilitation and Exercise for Solid Organ Transplant Optimal Recovery, a national network dedicated to achieving optimal well-being in transplant patients through exercise and rehabilitation. She is an investigator with the Canadian Donation and Transplantation Research Program and the co-lead for the research theme on restoring long-term health after transplantation.

Mara McAdams-DeMarco, Ph.D., M.S., is an associate professor of epidemiology and surgery on faculty at the Johns Hopkins University (JHU) School of Medicine. She has a joint appointment in the Department of Epidemiology at the Johns Hopkins Bloomberg School of Public Health. She is the director of clinical and outcomes research for the JHU Department of Surgery and Surgery Center for Outcomes Research. In these roles, she collaborates with many clinical faculty, including nephrologists, transplant surgeons, and geriatricians, across JHU and other universities. She has published more than 130 manuscripts, with more than half co-authored by trainees, and is the principal investigator (PI) of three National Institutes of Health–funded R01 studies. Her research focuses on the intersection of aging and end-stage renal disease, with a particular focus on older kidney transplant candidates and recipients. She conducted some of the first studies of frailty, delirium, cognitive function, and Alzheimer's disease among older kidney transplant patients. She is the PI of the oldest and largest cohort study of frailty among kidney transplant candidates and recipients and clinical trials of exercise interventions. Her career objectives are to better understand how novel aging metrics (frailty, cognitive function, physical function, and quality of life) can help improve risk prediction of adverse outcomes in older kidney transplant recipients and identify novel interventions to prevent adverse outcomes of aging.

Saeed Mohammad, M.D., M.S., cares for children with liver diseases, including those who may need a transplant. He has a great team who works hard to provide reassurance and care for both patients and their families during the stress of a critical illness, and he is extremely proud to work with them. Dr. Mohammad enjoys the long-term relationships that have developed with many of his patients and their families and is grateful to be a part of their lives. Dr. Mohammad's research is focused on improving the long-term outcomes and quality of life of children with chronic illnesses, particularly pediatric liver transplant recipients. His team is studying ways to improve their lives beyond standard medical therapy by measuring serum biomarkers and personalizing treatment.

Robert A. Montgomery, M.D., D.Phil., FACS, is the chairman and a professor of surgery at New York University (NYU) Langone Health and the director of the NYU Langone Transplant Institute. He received his M.D. with honors from the University of Rochester School of Medicine & Dentistry and D.Phil. in molecular immunology from Balliol College at the University of Oxford, England. Dr. Montgomery completed his general surgical training, multi-organ transplantation fellowship, and postdoctoral fellowship in human molecular genetics at Johns Hopkins University (JHU). For more than a decade, he served as the chief of transplant surgery and the director of the JHU Comprehensive Transplant Center. Dr. Montgomery was part of the team that developed the laparoscopic procedure for live kidney donation, a procedure that has become the standard throughout the world. He and the JHU team conceived the idea of the domino paired donation (kidney swaps) and the Hopkins protocol for desensitization of incompatible kidney transplant patients and performed the first chain of transplants started by an altruistic donor. He led the team that performed the first two-, three-, four-, five-, and six-way domino paired donations and eight-way multi-institutional domino paired donation, and he co-led the first 10-way open chain. He is credited in the 2010 *Guinness Book of World Records* with the most kidney transplants performed in 1 day. He is considered a world expert on kidney transplantation for highly sensitized and ABO incompatible patients and is referred the most complex patients from around the globe. Dr. Montgomery has had clinical and basic science research supported by the National Institutes of Health throughout his career. He has authored more than 300 peer-reviewed articles, has been cited more than 26,000 times, and has an H index of 84. His academic interests include HLA sensitization; tolerance protocols, including simultaneous solid organ and bone marrow transplantation; bio-artificial organs; and xenotransplantation. He has received important awards and distinctions, including a Fulbright Scholarship and a Thomas J. Watson Fellowship and memberships in the Phi Beta Kappa and Alpha Omega Alpha academic honor societies. He has been awarded multiple scholarships from the American College of Surgeons and the American Society of Transplant Surgeons. The National Kidney Foundation of Maryland recognized his contributions to the field of transplantation with the Champion of Hope Award, the National Kidney Registry with the Terasaki Medical Innovation Award, and the Greater New York Hospital Association with the Profile in Courage Award. He also received a heart transplant in 2018.

David Mulligan, M.D., FACS, is a professor and the chair of transplantation and immunology at Yale University, skilled in liver transplantation (especially living donor transplants), kidney and pancreas transplantation, hepatobiliary surgery, and immunology. Dr. Mulligan graduated from the University of Louisville School of Medicine. He was honored to build the Multiorgan Transplant Program at the Mayo Clinic in Arizona from 1998 to 2013, with outstanding growth in all solid organ transplantation with some of the best outcomes in the United States. He transformed the multi-organ transplant program at Yale to be one of the most innovative and academic institutions where patient-centered care can be met with cutting-edge research and science. He was recently elected the president of United Network for Organ Sharing/Organ Procurement and Transplantation Network and the chair of the Advisory Committee on Organ Transplantation to the Secretary of Health and Human Services to lead the oversight and policy development of organ transplantation in the United States. He also serves as the councilor at large for the board of governors of the American Association for the Study of Liver Diseases and the chair of the Business Practice Services Committee of the American Society of Transplant Surgeons. Dr. Mulligan is heavily involved in developing new policies and guidance across all organ transplantation and allocation during the COVID-19 pandemic for the safest possible outcomes for patients and providers alike.

Jignesh K. Patel, M.D., Ph.D., FACC, FRCP, FAST, FAHA, is a clinical professor of medicine, the medical director of heart transplant, the director of the Cardiac Amyloid Program, and the director of heart transplant research at Cedars-Sinai Smidt Heart Institute. His clinical and research interests focus on cardiac amyloidosis and transplant immunology. Dr. Patel serves on the Leadership Advisory Forum and is the past chair of the Heart Failure and Transplantation Council of the International Society for Heart and Lung Transplantation. He serves on the Heart Failure and Transplant Leadership Council at the American College of Cardiology. He is the associate editor of the *American Journal of Transplantation* and *Current Transplantation Reports*.

Tanjala S. Purnell, Ph.D., M.P.H., is an epidemiologist and health services researcher with more than a decade of research experience related to identifying and addressing patient/family, health care system, and community factors influencing health and health care disparities for adults with cardiovascular disease risk factors, including hypertension, chronic kidney disease, and diabetes. She is an assistant professor of cardiovascular disease and clinical epidemiology at the Johns Hopkins Bloomberg School of Public Health. She holds joint faculty appointments in the Johns Hopkins University Departments of Surgery, Health Policy and Management, and Health, Behavior and Society. In her role as an associate director of the Johns Hopkins Urban Health Institute, Dr. Purnell co-leads the institute's efforts to facilitate and recognize collaborations among communities, universities, health care delivery systems, government, and the private sector to build collective capacity for achieving health equity in Baltimore. She is also the associate director for education and training at the Johns Hopkins Center for Health Equity, where she leads the center's award-winning educational and training programs for public health, nursing, and medical scholars working to advance health equity. She is the director of community and stakeholder engagement for the Johns Hopkins Epidemiology Research Group in Organ Transplantation; core faculty at the Welch Center for Prevention, Epidemiology, and Clinical Research; and affiliated faculty with the Bloomberg American Health Initiative and the Center for Health Services and Outcomes Research. Nationally, Dr. Purnell is the chair of the American Society of Transplant Surgeons' Diversity, Equity, and Inclusion Committee, and she previously served as the Region 2 representative to the United Network for Organ Sharing/Organ Procurement and Transplantation Network Minority Affairs Committee. She is a native of the Mississippi Delta and an alumna of Tougaloo College, where she obtained her B.S. in computer science. Dr. Purnell has received several national and international research honors and published findings from her work in leading medical and public health journals, including *JAMA*, *Health Affairs*, the *Journal of the American Society of Nephrology*, the *American Journal of Hypertension*, the *American Journal of Transplantation*, and *Diabetes Care*. She is deeply committed to community engagement, teaching, and mentoring, and she speaks often on the impact of COVID-19 and systemic racism on existing health and health care disparities in the United States. She is also the recipient of multiple Teaching Excellence Awards from the Johns Hopkins Bloomberg School of Public Health.

Eyal Shemesh, M.D., is the chief of the Division of Behavioral and Developmental Pediatrics at the Kravis Children's Hospital and a professor in the Departments of Pediatrics and Psychiatry at the Icahn School of Medicine at Mount Sinai. Dr. Shemesh trained in the Mount Sinai "Triple Board" program as a pediatrician, psychiatrist, and a child psychiatrist.

Since graduating from that program, he has been continuously funded by federal and philanthropic entities to conduct research in the interface between psychiatric/behavioral and medical disorders, with nonadherence as the important outcome, in children and adults. Among other areas of research concentration, Dr. Shemesh and his group discovered, studied, and developed the use of variation in medication blood levels as a marker of nonadherence (the Medication Level Variability Index) in transplant recipients and have been studying the impact of traumatic stress symptoms on several groups of chronically ill patients, including transplant recipients. In addition to this research work, Dr. Shemesh has created and has been directing specialty programs that enhance patients' access to mental health care by integrating mental health concepts into the work of specialty and primary care clinics in pediatric and adult practices.

Charlie Thomas, M.S.W., LCSW, ACSW, FNKF, received his M.S.W. from Arizona State University in 1980 and his B.A. in 1979 from San Diego State University, where he graduated with distinction in social welfare. He is a licensed clinical social worker in Arizona and a member of the National Association of Social Workers' Academy of Certified Social Workers. He has been employed as a transplant social worker with the Banner-University Medical Center in Phoenix, Arizona, since 1985 and was the dialysis/transplant consultant for the Salt River Pima-Maricopa Indian Community (1998–2012). He provides direct services to liver, kidney, and pancreas transplant patients and living kidney and liver donors. He also provided consultation regarding chronic kidney disease, including dialysis, transplantation, and organ donation with American Indians. Mr. Thomas has served with many national and regional organizations, including the American Society for Transplantation Public Policy Committee; the National Kidney Foundation (NKF) board of directors and as a national chairperson of its Council of Nephrology Social Workers and Public Policy Task Force; the NKF of Arizona board of directors since 1988 and several affiliate committees; the medical review board of the Intermountain End-Stage Renal Disease Network; United Network for Organ Sharing Patient Affairs Committee, Task Force on Access to Transplantation, and the chairperson of the Social Work Advisory Task Force; the National Living Donor Consensus Conference; and the Arizona Coalition on Donation as the president. In 1999, Mr. Thomas was an expert advisor to the Institute of Medicine regarding the proposed Final Rule for the Organ Procurement and Transplantation Network. In 2000, the governor of Arizona appointed him to the State Rehabilitation Council, where he was the chair from 2003 to 2005. In 2007, the Centers for Medicare & Medicaid Services recruited Mr. Thomas to train its surveyors on the psychosocial issues of organ transplant recipients and living donors. He teaches social welfare policy and community practice to graduate and undergraduate social work students at Arizona State University. He has authored many articles and presented at many national conferences and meetings. He has organized a coalition of transplant hospitals and nonprofit health associations to promote living donor leave for Arizona State employees, and in 2008, the Arizona legislature passed relevant legislation signed by the governor. His awards include the Health Care Heroes Award—Non-Physician by the *Phoenix Business Journal* (2006), the Robert W. Whitlock Lifetime Achievement Award from the NKF Council of Nephrology Social Workers (2015), and the Clinician of Distinction Award from the American Society of Transplantation (2020).

Fanny Vlahos, J.D., L.L.B., is a patient with cystic fibrosis (CF) who underwent a double lung transplant in 2012, when her son was only 10 months old. She is a licensed attorney (Illinois) and holds degrees in American and Canadian law and an undergraduate degree in English language and literature, with honors. In recent years, Ms. Vlahos has used her unique position to champion access to quality health care and is involved with the CF Foundation on the Clinical Care Guidelines Committee, Lung Transplant Initiative, and Steering Committee, among others. She has dedicated her efforts to public policy advocacy at both the state and national levels.

Kirsten Wentlandt, M.D., Ph.D., M.HSc., is a palliative care physician from the University of Toronto, the W. Gifford-Jones Professor in Pain Control and Palliative Care, and the head of the Division of Palliative Care. Her clinical work and research are focused on nonmalignant palliative care populations, with ambulatory clinics supporting advanced lung, heart, pulmonary hypertension, and transplant populations. She also works with various national, provincial, and regional committees that focus on developing strategies to improve access to quality palliative care for all patients.